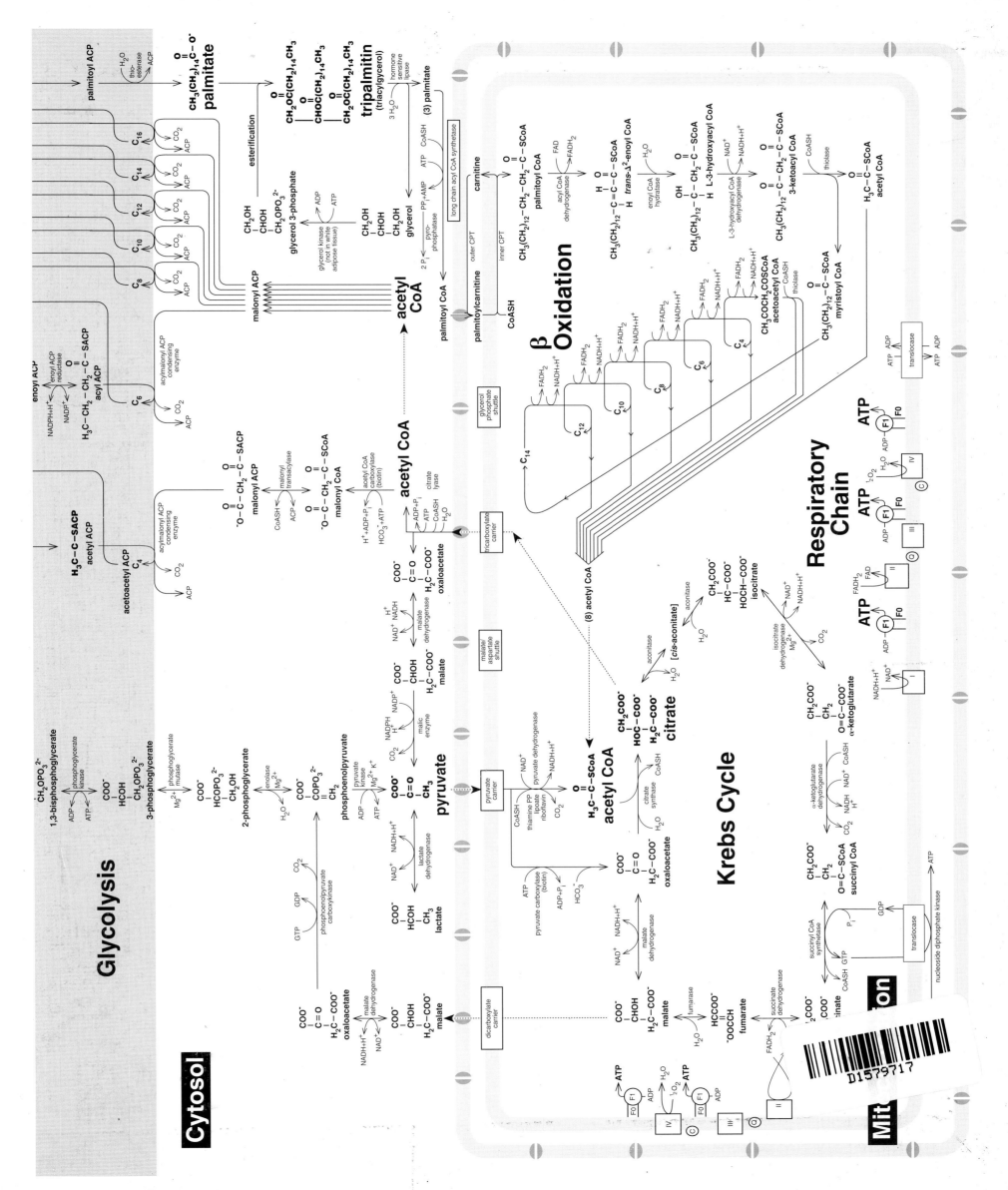

Metabolism at a Glance

J. G. Salway BSc, MSc, PhD
Senior Lecturer in Medical Biochemistry
School of Biological Sciences
University of Surrey
Guildford GU2 5XH

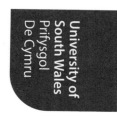
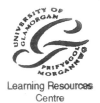

Learning Resources
Centre

OXFORD
BLACKWELL SCIENTIFIC PUBLICATIONS
LONDON EDINBURGH BOSTON
MELBOURNE PARIS BERLIN VIENNA

© 1994 by Blackwell Scientific Publications
Editorial Offices:
Osney Mead, Oxford OX2 0EL
25 John Street, London WC1N 2BL
23 Ainslie Place, Edinburgh EH3 6AJ
238 Main Street, Cambridge
　　Massachusetts 02142, USA
54 University Street, Carlton
　　Victoria 3053, Australia

Other Editorial Offices:
Librairie Arnette SA
1, rue de Lille
75007 Paris
France

Blackwell Wissenschafts-Verlag GmbH
Düsseldorfer Str. 38
D-10707 Berlin
Germany

Blackwell MZV
Feldgasse 13
A-1238 Wien
Austria

First published 1994

Set by Steve Meyfroidt using Quark Xpress 3.11
on an Apple Macintosh computer and
output in Malaysia by Expo Holdings Sdn Bhd
on a Linotron 300 phototypesetter
Printed and bound in Great Britain
at the University Press, Cambridge

DISTRIBUTORS

Marston Book Services Ltd
PO Box 87
Oxford OX2 0DT
(*Orders:* Tel: 0865 791155
　　　　　 Fax: 0865 791927
　　　　　 Telex: 837515)

USA
Blackwell Scientific Publications, Inc.
238 Main Street
Cambridge, MA 02142
(*Orders:* Tel: 800 759-6102
　　　　　 617 876-7000)

Canada
Times Mirror Professional Publishing, Ltd
130 Flaska Drive
Markham, Ontario L6G 1B8
(*Orders:* Tel: 800 268-4178
　　　　　 416 470-6739)

Australia
Blackwell Scientific Publications Pty Ltd
54 University Street
Carlton, Victoria 3053
(*Orders:* Tel: 03 347-5552)

A catalogue record for this title
is available from the British Library

ISBN   0-632-03258-8 (BSP)
　　　　 0-632-03422-X (Four Dragons)

Library of Congress
Cataloging in Publication Data

Salway, J. G.
　　Metabolism at a glance / J.G. Salway
　　　　　 p.　　　cm.
　　Includes bibliographical references
　　and index.
　　ISBN 0-632-03258-8.
　　ISBN 0-632-03422-X (Four Dragons)
　　1. Metabolism.　 I. Title.
　　[DNLM: 1. Metabolism.
　　QU 120 S186m 1994]
　　QP171.S1185　 1994
　　616.3′9—dc20
　　DNLM/DLC
　　for Library of Congress

Contents

Preface

The need for a concise, introductory book on intermediary metabolism became apparent to me in the early 1970s during tutorials with small groups of first year science and medical students who were wrestling with this complicated subject. The educational problem seemed to stem from the way in which metabolism was presented. The first exposure to junior school pupils was, of necessity, very basic and virtually unrecognizable from the quantum leaps in complexity needed by sixth-formers and then by university students. At each level of progress, the simplifications of the previous level were overruled. Moreover the textbooks covered the various pathways individually and were only partly successful at integrating the various metabolic processes of fat, protein, and carbohydrate metabolism. There was a need for a text on metabolism which spanned the transitions from the sixth-form, through to university first-year science and preclinical biochemistry studies, and on to more advanced topics emphasizing the medical relevance of biochemistry. Furthermore, these transitions needed to be gradual, allowing students to absorb detail as their education progressed in a format which retained its familiarity and permitted continual integration of the pathways.

Thus the concept was developed for a concise book based on a series of two-page spreads. Each spread covers a particular topic but is based on a repeating series of detailed metabolic charts on which the principal features of the metabolic pathway are highlighted. The early huge, hand-drawn maps were appreciated in tutorials, and I was also encouraged by positive feedback and support from Mr John Luxton, then of Lawnswood School now Head of Science at Ralph Thoresby School, Leeds. However, a solution to the technical complexities of producing such a book had to await the computerized technologies of the 1990s.

The result is a book designed as a companion to the many excellent biochemistry textbooks. It provides a concise synopsis of the principal metabolic pathways involved in mammalian intermediary metabolism. Selection of the subject matter has been dictated largely by the need to suit the two-page-spread format of the book; inevitably, this has caused certain topics to be omitted. This simplified, didactic, cartographical approach is designed to guide students through the maze of metabolic pathways and their interrelationships. My intention is that the format should aid both tutorial teaching and individual revision.

The book, like a geographical map, can be used at different levels of complexity. The reader can choose to zoom along the main motorways of metabolism to gain an overview of the subject. Alternatively, the reader can focus on details of particular interest. Some of the early chapters will be of interest to students of A-level biology and similar courses. Such students who progress to study the biological and medical sciences at university will grow into this book throughout their undergraduate studies. The book will also be a handy reference work for senior biological and medical scientists and researchers who need to refresh 'at a glance' their knowledge and understanding of metabolic pathways.

Finally, a comment on the choice of biochemical nomenclature. Since this text is a 'companion book', it seemed logical to adopt the nomenclature of its famous companions. However, this revealed considerable diversity from international convention. For example, 2-oxoglutarate (IUPAC approved) is rarely used and has yet to replace the traditional α-ketoglutarate; although the hybrid compromise α-oxoglutarate appears in at least one text. Because of this confusion, I have kept mainly to the traditional nomenclature to match the principal student textbooks in biochemistry.

Acknowledgements

It is a pleasure to record the help and encouragement provided by so many people during the long gestation period of this book. In particular, my colleagues Dr Keith Snell and Gordon Hartman have always given generously of their time and advice on many occasions. Invaluable help with checking, and specialist advice on the text and subject matter, have been provided by the following: Prof. P. Cohen, Dr J. Chakraborty, Dr G. W. Gould, Prof. G. G. Gibson, Prof. J. L. Harwood, Dr R. H. Hinton, Dr S. S. Klioze, Dr D. F. V. Lewis, Prof. V. Marks, Dr T. Pepper, Dr G. Robbins, Dr H. S. A. Sherratt, Mr C. J. Smith, Ms T. D. Spurway, Dr B. C. Stace, Dr P. B. Stace, Dr J. C. M. Stewart, Dr C. M. Williams and Dr H. Wood. Over the years, many students have contributed and influenced this book in many ways, in particular Ms A. Blackburn and Ms R. Bains who have read the manuscript and provided constructive advice from a student's perspective. My appreciation is also extended to all those at Blackwell Scientific Publications who have at all times dealt patiently with the inevitable problems; especially Dr S. Taylor, Mr E. Wates and Ms Mary Fox. The tasks of reducing my (literally) man-size original of the metabolic chart to book size, interpreting my sketches, and integrating the text with the artwork, were done by Mr Steve Meyfroidt. He remained invariably cheerful and helpful in spite of the need for tedious revisions. For all of this, I am most grateful. My son Andrew typed the manuscript, my wife Nicky took over the gardening, and my daughter Katherine (whose room is next to my study), obliged by moderating the volume and choice of her music when I was writing.

Finally, the responsibility for any errors, ambiguities and omissions is of course mine, and advice and comments from readers would be most welcome.

Further reading

Devlin T. M. Ed. (1992) *Textbook of Biochemistry with Clinical Correlations*. Wiley-Liss, New York (1185 pp).

Hardie D. G. (1992) *Biochemical Messengers*. Chapman & Hall, London (311 pp).

Horton H. R., Moran L. A., Ochs R. S., Rawn J. D. & Scrimgeour K. G. (1993) *Principles of Biochemistry*. Neil Patterson Publishers/Prentice Hall, Englewood Cliffs, NJ.

Martin B. R. (1987) *Metabolic Regulation*. Blackwell Scientific Publications, Oxford (299 pp).

Murray R. K., Granner D. K., Mayes P. A. & Rodwell V. W. (1993) *Harper's Biochemistry*, 23rd edn. Appleton & Lange, Norwalk, Connecticut (806 pp).

Stryer L. (1986) *Biochemistry*, 3rd edn. W. H. Freeman and Company, New York (1089 pp).

Voet D. & Voet J. G. (1990) *Biochemistry*. Wiley, New York (1223 pp).

Introduction to metabolic pathways

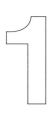

Chart 1 opposite. Map of the main pathways of intermediary metabolism.

Metabolic charts

The metabolic map opposite will, at first sight, appear to most readers to be a confusing, incomprehensible jumble of chemical formulae. There can be no doubt that metabolic charts **are** complex, and many biochemists remember their own first introduction to metabolism as a somewhat bewildering experience.

The first important thing to remember is that the chart is no more than a form of map. In many respects it is similar to a map of the London Underground which is also very complicated (see Diagram 1.1 below). With the latter, however, we have learned to suppress the overwhelming detail in order to concentrate on those aspects relevant to a particular journey. For example, if asked "How would you get from Archway to Queensway?" the reply is likely to be: "Take the Northern Line travelling south to Tottenham Court Road, then change to the Central Line travelling west to Queensway". An equally valid answer would be: "Enter Archway station, buy a ticket at the kiosk, pass through the ticket inspector's barrier and proceed to the platform. When a train arrives, enter and remain seated as it passes through Tuffnell Park, Kentish Town, Camden Town, Euston, Warren Street and Goode Street. When it reaches Tottenham Court Road, stand up and leave the train, transfer to platform 1..., etc., etc...." Each of these details, although essential for completion of the journey, is not necessary to an **overall** understanding of the journey.

A similar approach should be used when studying the metabolic chart. The details of individual enzyme reactions are very complex and very important. Many biochemists, including some of the world's most famous, have been researching individual enzymes such as **phosphofructokinase-1**, **pyruvate dehydrogenase** and **glucokinase** for many years. The detailed properties of these important enzymes and the mechanism of their reactions are superbly summarized in several standard biochemistry textbooks. However, these details should not be allowed to confuse the mind of the reader when asked the question: 'How is glucose metabolized to fat?'. When faced with such a problem, the student should learn to recall sufficient detail relevant to an overall understanding of the pathways involved, while at the same time maintaining an awareness of the detailed background information and mechanisms.

Chart 1: Subcellular distribution of metabolic pathways

The metabolic chart opposite shows how certain pathways are located in the **cytosol** of the cell, whereas others are located in the **mitochondrion**. Certain other enzymes are associated with subcellular structures such as the **endoplasmic reticulum**, for example **glucose 6-phosphatase**. Others are associated with organelles such as the nucleus and peroxisomes which, for simplicity, are not shown in the chart.

The enzymes required to catalyse the reactions in the various metabolic pathways are organized among the different subcellular compartments within the cell. For example, the enzymes involved in **fatty acid synthesis**, the **pentose phosphate pathway** and **glycolysis** are nearly all located in the **cytosol**. As we can see, most of the reactions involved in harnessing energy for the cell, the **Krebs cycle**, **β-oxidation** and **respiratory chain**, are located in the **mitochondrion**, which is frequently called 'the power house of the cell'.

Mitochondrion—(plural, mitochondria)

Most animal and plant cells contain mitochondria. An important exception in most animal species is the mature red blood cell. Mitochondria are usually sausage-shaped organelles. They are surrounded by a double system of membranes conveniently described as the **outer membrane** and the **inner membrane** which separate an **intermembrane space**. Interestingly, they contain ribosomes for protein synthesis, some of their own genes, and reproduce by binary fission. In short, they are largely autonomous and biologists have suggested that they were originally bacterial cells which have evolved a symbiotic relationship with a larger cell. They have therefore been described as 'cells within a cell'.

The outer membrane of the mitochondrion is fairly typical of most cell membranes, being composed of 50% protein and 50% lipids. It contains a channel-forming protein called **porin**, which renders it permeable to molecules of less than 10000 daltons. This is in contrast to the inner membrane, which forms one of the most impermeable barriers within the cell. This inner membrane contains 80% protein and 20% lipid, and is folded inwards to form cristae (not shown), which project into the matrix. It is, however, permeable to water and gases such as oxygen. Also, certain metabolites can cross the inner membrane, but only when assisted by carrier systems such as the **dicarboxylate carrier**.

When sections of the inner membrane are stained for electron microscopy, mushroom-like projections, the F_0/F_1 **particles** appear. These are respiratory particles which are thought to be embedded in the membrane *in vivo*, but which following fixation project into the matrix. These particles are involved in **adenosine triphosphate (ATP)** synthesis by oxidative phosphorylation, and are functionally associated with the respiratory chain.

The **matrix** of the mitochondrion contains the enzymes of the **β-oxidation** pathway and also most of the enzymes needed for the **Krebs cycle**. An important exception is **succinate dehydrogenase**, which is linked to the **respiratory chain** in the inner membrane. Certain mitochondria have special enzymes, for example, liver mitochondria contain the enzymes necessary for ketogenesis (see Chapter 34) and urea synthesis (see Chapter 16).

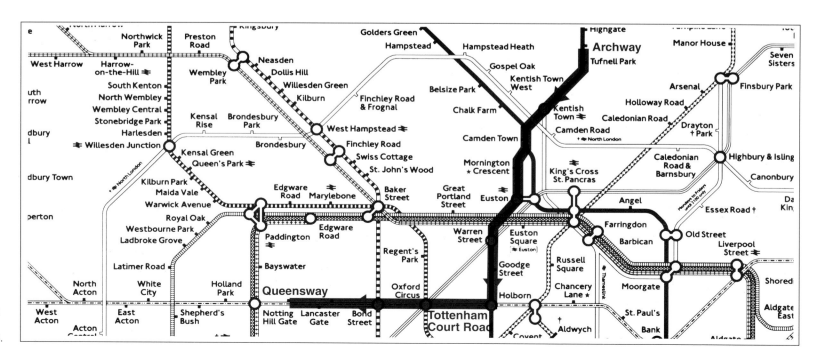

Diagram 1.1. Map of the London Underground with permission. LRT Registered User No. 93/1726.

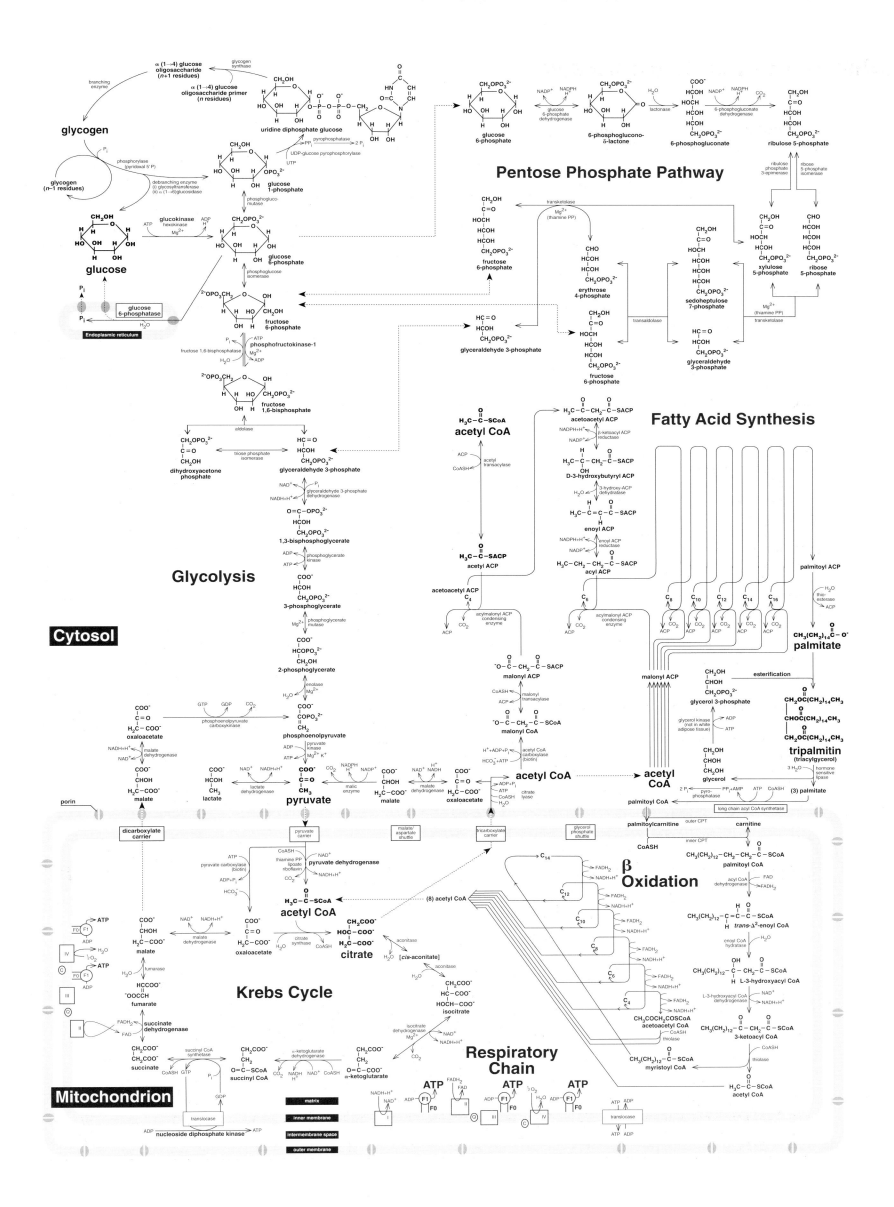

Biosynthesis of ATP, part I. ATP: the molecule that powers metabolism

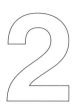

Chart 2 opposite. The biosynthesis of ATP.

How living cells conserve energy in a biologically useful form

A lump of coal can be burned in a power station to generate electricity, which is a very useful and versatile form of energy. Apart from coal, several other fuels, such as oil, peat and even public refuse can be used to generate electricity. This electrical energy can then be used to power innumerable industrial machines and domestic appliances, which are essential to our modern way of life.

Living cells have a similarly versatile energy resource in the molecule, adenosine triphosphate (**ATP**). ATP can be generated by oxidizing several metabolic fuels, although carbohydrates and fats are especially important. ATP is used in innumerable vital metabolic reactions and physiological functions, not only in humans, but in all forms of life. The primary objective of intermediary metabolism is to maintain a steady supply of ATP so that living cells can grow, reproduce, and respond to the stresses and strains imposed by starvation, exercise, overeating, etc.

The ATP molecule has two phosphoanhydride bonds which provide the energy for life

The ATP molecule has two phosphoanhydride bonds which, when hydrolysed at physiological pH, release 7.3 kCal (30.66 kJ) as energy which can be used for metabolic purposes. These two phosphoanhydride bonds were referred to by Lipmann in 1941 as 'high-energy' bonds. However, this term is a misleading concept which (apologies apart) has nearly been banished from the textbooks. In fact, these phosphoanhydride bonds are in no way different from any other covalent bonds.

Adenosine triphosphate (ATP)

Chart 2: The biosynthesis of ATP

We will see later (Chapter 5) how glucose is oxidized and energy is conserved as ATP. ATP can be synthesized by phosphorylation of adenosine diphosphate (ADP) by two types of process. One does not need oxygen and is known as **substrate-level phosphorylation**. The other requires oxygen and is known as **oxidative phosphorylation**.

Substrate-level phosphorylation

Examination of the chart opposite shows that two reactions in glycolysis, namely the **phosphoglycerate kinase** and **pyruvate kinase** reactions, produce ATP by direct phosphorylation of ADP. This is **substrate-level phosphorylation** and is especially important for generating ATP if the tissues are inadequately supplied with oxygen.

Another example of substrate-level phosphorylation occurs in the Krebs cycle. The reaction, catalysed by **succinyl CoA synthetase**, produces **GTP** (guanosine triphosphate), which is structurally similar to ATP. The enzyme **nucleoside diphosphate kinase** catalyses the conversion of GTP to ATP.

Oxidative phosphorylation

In the presence of oxygen, oxidative phosphorylation is by far the most important mechanism for synthesizing ATP. This process is coupled to the oxidation of the reduced 'hydrogen carriers' $NADH+H^+$ and $FADH_2$ via the respiratory chain.

The "hydrogen carriers" NAD⁺ and FAD
NAD⁺ (nicotinamide adenine dinucleotide)

NAD^+ is a hydrogen carrier derived from the vitamin niacin. It is a coenzyme involved in several oxidation/reduction reactions catalysed by dehydrogenases. In the example opposite, taken from Krebs cycle, **malate dehydrogenase** catalyses the oxidation of malate to oxaloacetate. During this reaction, NAD^+ is reduced to form $NADH+H^+$, which is oxidized by the respiratory chain and three molecules of ATP are formed.

FAD (flavin adenine dinucleotide)

FAD is a hydrogen carrier derived from the vitamin riboflavin. It differs from NAD^+ in that it is covalently bound to its dehydrogenase enzyme, and is therefore known as a prosthetic group. In the example opposite the **succinate dehydrogenase** reaction is shown with FAD being reduced to $FADH_2$. Succinate dehydrogenase is bound to the inner membrane of the mitochondrion and is an integral part of the respiratory chain. When $FADH_2$ is oxidized by this process, a total of two ATP molecules are formed.

ATP / ADP translocase

The inner membrane of the mitochondrion is impermeable to ATP. A protein complex known as the 'ATP/ADP translocase' is needed for the export of ATP in return for the import of ADP (adenosine diphosphate) and P_i (inorganic phosphate).

Reference

Carusi E.A., It's time we replaced 'high-energy phosphate group' with 'phosphoryl group'. *Biochem Ed*, **20**, 145–147, 1992.

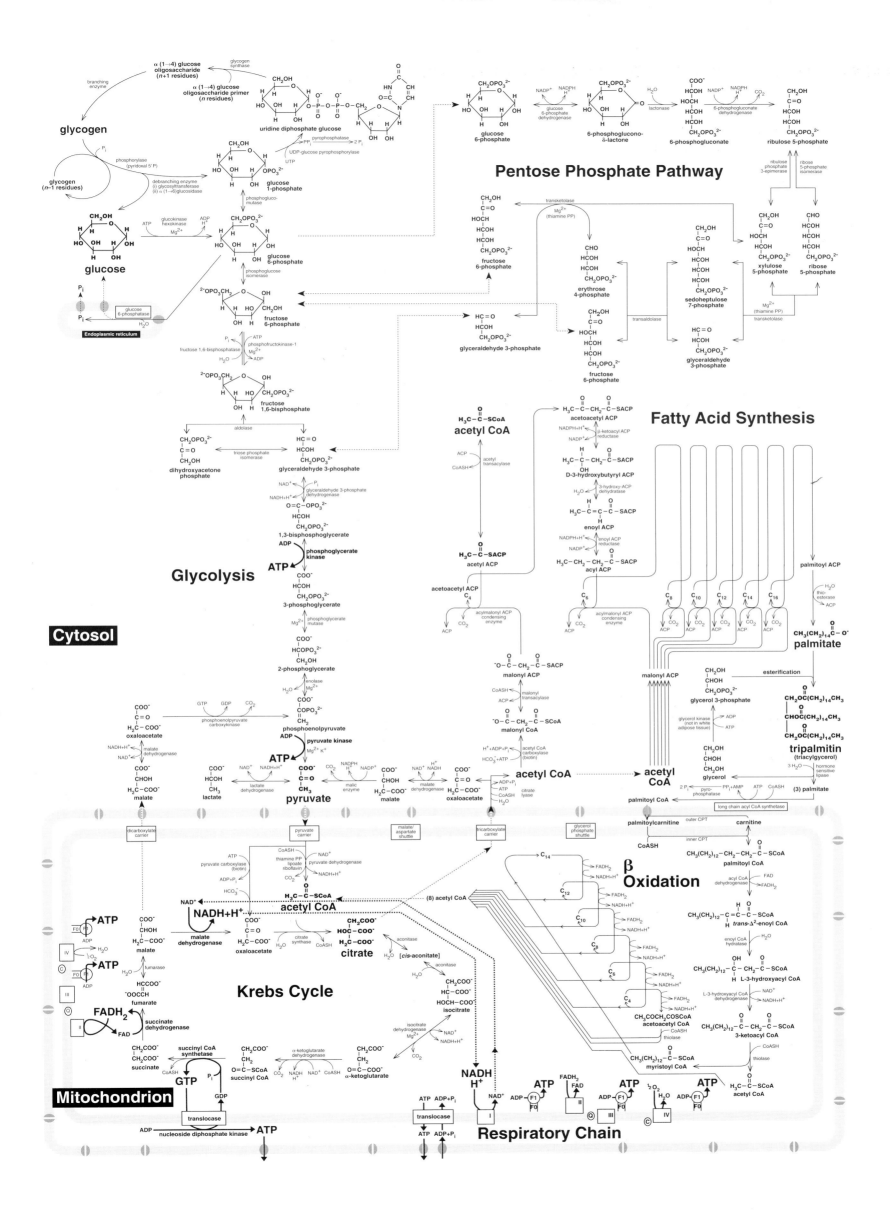

Biosynthesis of ATP, part II: the respiratory chain, and inhibitors and uncouplers of oxidative phosphorylation

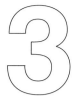

Respiratory chain

The respiratory chain (Diagrams 3.1 and 3.2) comprises complexes I (NADH-ubiquinone reductase), II (succinate-ubiquinone reductase), III (ubiquinol-cytochrome C reductase) and IV (cytochrome C oxidase). These are linked by ubiquinone (Q) and cytochrome C. The latter are mobile molecules which diffuse through the membrane. Q serves to shuttle electrons from complexes I and II to complex III. Similarly, cytochrome C shuttles electrons from complex III to complex IV. The synthesis of ATP via the respiratory chain is the result of two coupled processes: electron transport and oxidative phosphorylation.

Electron transport (Diagram 3.1)

This involves the oxidation (i.e. the removal of electrons) from $NADH+H^+$,

or $FADH_2$ with transport of the electrons through the chain until they are donated to molecular oxygen, which is consequently reduced to water.

Oxidative phosphorylation and proton transport (Diagram 3.2)

According to Mitchell's chemiosmotic hypothesis, the electron transport just described drives proton pumps in complexes I, III and IV by a mechanism which is not understood. This causes an increased concentration of protons in the intermembrane space. As the protons return through the F_0 particle (the proton channel) they activate the F_1 particle (F_1 ATP synthetase) to phosphorylate ADP to form ATP.

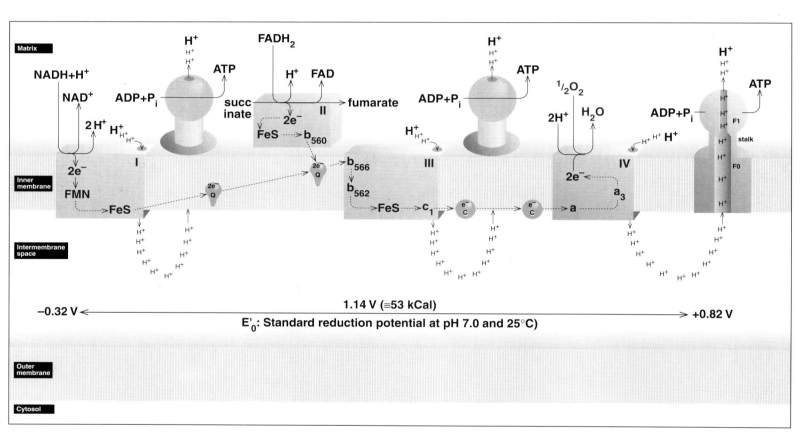

Diagram 3.1. The respiratory chain showing the flow of electrons from $NADH+H^+$ and $FADH_2$ to oxygen, with the formation of water.

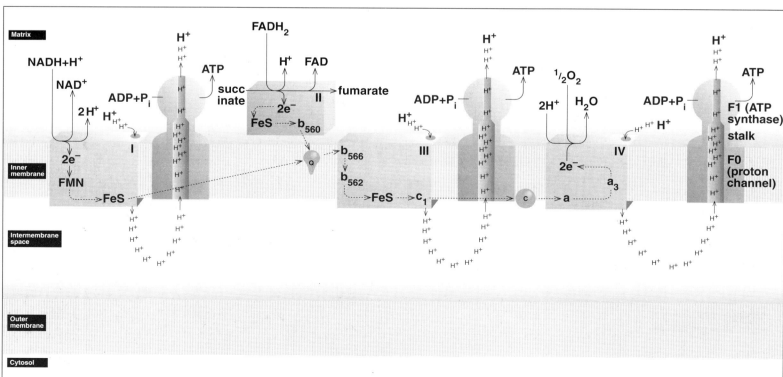

Diagram 3.2. The respiratory chain showing the extrusion of protons into the intermembrane space. As the protons return via the F_0 channel, the F_1 unit forms ATP from ADP.

Inhibitors of the respiratory chain

The use of compounds that inhibit or interact with the respiratory chain has contributed to our understanding of the mechanism of this process. These compounds (see Diagram 3.3), can be organized into three groups: those that inhibit the flow of electrons; those that interfere with the flow of protons; and miscellaneous compounds.

Interference with the flow of electrons
Rotenone and amytal
Ubiquinone (Q), which is a mobile component of the inner membrane, shuttles to and fro between complexes I and III, and in so doing transports electrons from complex I to complex III. Rotenone and amytal prevent the transfer of electrons from complex I to ubiquinone.

Carboxin
Ubiquinone can also shuttle electrons from complex II to complex III. Carboxin prevents the transfer of electrons from complex II to ubiquinone.

Malonate
Malonate, by virtue of its structural similarity to succinate, is a competitive inhibitor of succinate dehydrogenase, which is a component of complex II.

Antimycin A and myxothiazol
Cytochrome C, which is loosely associated with the outer face of the inner membrane, shuttles electrons from complex III to complex IV. The transfer of electrons from complex III to cytochrome C is inhibited by antimycin A, and even more potently by myxothiazol.

Cyanide, carbon monoxide and azide
Electrons are transferred from complex IV to molecular oxygen. This process is inhibited by cyanide, carbon monoxide and azide.

Interference with the flow of protons
Oligomycin and dicyclohexylcarbodiimide (DCCD)
These compounds block the proton channel of the F_0 particle. Consequently, the flux of protons needed for ATP synthesis by the F_1 particle is prevented.

2,4-dinitrophenol (DNP)
Dinitrophenol is a weak acid. Therefore its base 2,4-dinitrophenate accepts H^+, producing the undissociated acid form 2,4-dinitrophenol, which is lipophilic and able to diffuse across the inner mitochondrial membrane. This leakage of H^+ caused by DNP reduces the flux of H^+ through the F_0F_1 particle, thereby preventing ATP synthesis. However, the flow of electrons is unrestricted by DNP and its effect is described as 'uncoupling ATP synthesis from electron transport'.

Carbonylcyanide-p-trifluoromethoxyphenylhydrazone (FCCP)
Whereas DNP is the classic uncoupler, it is now outclassed by FCCP. This is a lipophilic, weak acid like DNP, but is a more effective uncoupler of oxidative phosphorylation.

Some other compounds that affect the respiratory chain
Tetramethyl-p-phenyldiamine (TMPD)
TMPD is an artificial electron donor that can transfer electrons to cytochrome C. Since ascorbate can reduce TMPD, these compounds can be used experimentally to study the respiratory chain.

Bongkrekic acid
Bongkrekic acid (a toxic contaminant of bongkrek, which is a food prepared from coconuts) inhibits the ATP/ADP translocase and therefore prevents the export of ATP and the import of ADP. Bongkrekic acid binds to the inner aspect of the ATP/ADP translocase.

Atractyloside
Atractyloside has a similar effect to bongkrekic acid, except that it inhibits from the outer aspect of the ATP/ADP translocase.

Diagram 3.3. Inhibitors, uncouplers and other compounds that affect the respiratory chain.

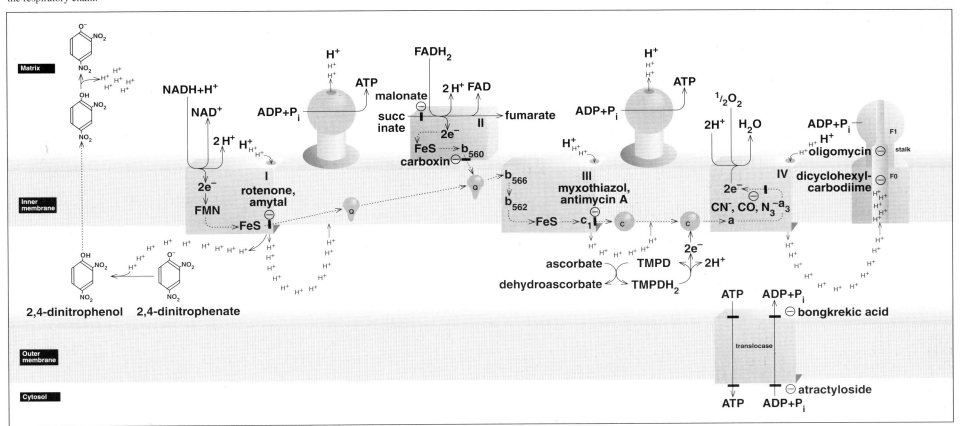

The oxidation of cytosolic NADH+H⁺: the malate/aspartate shuttle, and the glycerol phosphate shuttle

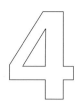

Oxidation of cytosolic NADH+H⁺

The **glycerol 3-phosphate dehydrogenase** reaction occurs in the cytosol and forms NADH+H⁺, which can be oxidized by the respiratory chain in the mitochondrion to produce ATP. However, molecules of NADH+H⁺ are unable to cross the inner membrane of the mitochondrion. This paradox is overcome by two mechanisms which enable 'reducing equivalents' to be transferred from the cytosol to the mitochondrion. They are the **malate/aspartate shuttle** and the **glycerol phosphate shuttle**.

Chart 4.1 opposite. The malate/aspartate shuttle.

The malate/aspartate shuttle

This shuttle (opposite page) starts with cytosolic **oxaloacetate.** First, **cytosolic malate dehydrogenase** uses the NADH+H⁺ to reduce oxaloacetate to malate. The latter is transported into the mitochondrial matrix in exchange for α-ketoglutarate. Here it is oxidized by malate dehydrogenase back to oxaloacetate, and the NADH+H⁺ released is available for oxidative phosphorylation by the respiratory chain, producing **three** molecules of ATP.

The oxaloacetate must now be returned to the cytosol. The problem is that it too is unable to cross the inner mitochondrial membrane. Accordingly, it is transformed to **aspartate** in a reaction catalysed by aspartate aminotransferase. Aspartate leaves the mitochondrion via the glutamate/aspartate carrier in exchange for glutamate. Once in the cytosol, aspartate is transaminated by aspartate aminotransferase, and thus oxaloacetate is restored to the cytosol, thereby completing the cycle.

The glycerol phosphate shuttle

This shuttle (below), which is particularly important in insects, uses the cytosolic NADH+H⁺ in the presence of **glycerol 3-phosphate dehydrogenase** to reduce **dihydroxyacetone phosphate** to form **glycerol 3-phosphate**. The latter diffuses into the intermembrane space of the mitochondrion. Here it is oxidized by the mitochondrial glycerol 3-phosphate dehydrogenase isoenzyme, which is associated with the outer surface of the inner membrane. The products of the reaction are dihydroxyacetone phosphate (which diffuses back into the cytosol) and FADH₂. This FADH₂ can be oxidized by the respiratory chain but, since it donates its electrons to ubiquinone (Q), only **two** molecules of ATP are produced.

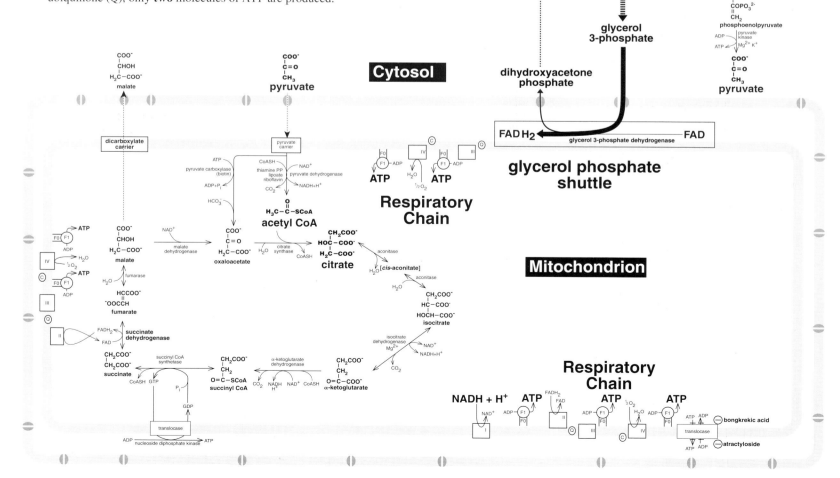

Chart 4.2. The glycerol phosphate shuttle.

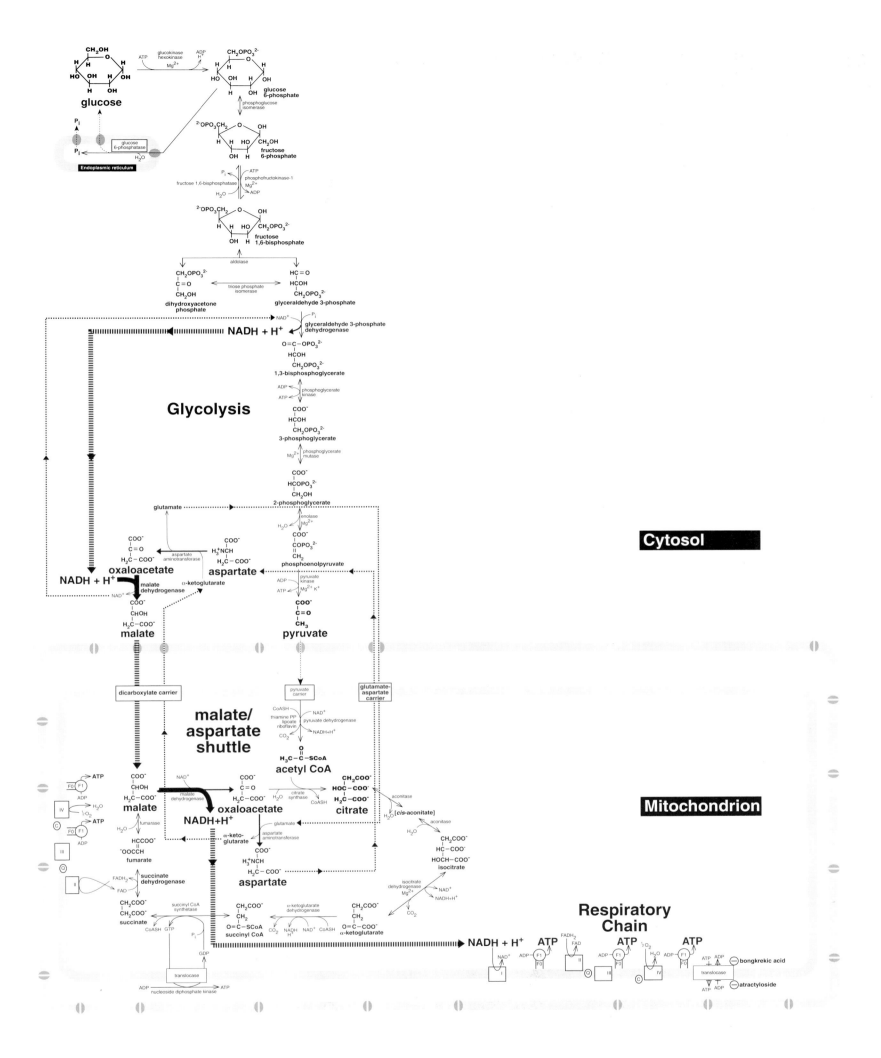

Metabolism of glucose to give energy

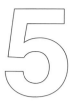

Chart 5 opposite. Metabolism of glucose to give energy.

The glucose molecule, which is a rich store of chemical energy, burns vigorously in air to form carbon dioxide and water, and in the process energy escapes as heat. This can be represented by the following equation:

$$C_6H_{12}O_6 + 6\,O_2 \longrightarrow 6\,CO_2 + 6\,H_2O + \text{energy as heat}$$

glucose · oxygen · carbon dioxide · water

Carbohydrate-containing foods such as starch are digested to glucose, which is then absorbed into the blood, and it is well known that 'glucose gives you energy'. Bearing in mind that the laws of thermodynamics apply to both animate and inanimate systems, we must now consider how living cells can release energy from a glucose molecule in a controlled way, so that the cell neither bursts into flames nor explodes in the process.

Once a glucose molecule has passed from the bloodstream into a cell, it is gradually transformed and dismantled in a controlled sequence of some two dozen biochemical steps, in a manner analogous to a production line in a factory. The several biochemical transformations are assisted by enzymes, some of which need cofactors supplied by vitamins to function properly. Such a series of biochemical reactions is known as a metabolic pathway.

Chart 5: glucose metabolism

The chart shows that, in order to conserve the energy from glucose as ATP, three metabolic pathways are involved. First, glucose is oxidized through the pathway known as **glycolysis**. The end product of glycolysis, two molecules of **pyruvate**, are then fed into the **Krebs cycle**, where they are completely oxidized to form six molecules of carbon dioxide. In the process, the hydrogen carriers NAD$^+$ and FAD, which are compounds incorporating the vitamins niacin and riboflavin respectively, become reduced to NADH+H$^+$ and FADH$_2$ and carry hydrogen to the **respiratory chain**. Here, energy is conserved in **ATP** molecules, while the hydrogen is eventually used to reduce oxygen to water (see Chapter 3).

The energy released from ATP on hydrolysis can then be used for biological work such as muscle contraction, protein synthesis and conduction of nerve impulses.

Several vitamins provide cofactors for the enzymes involved in these metabolic pathways. For example, the pyruvate dehydrogenase reaction needs niacin, thiamine, riboflavin, lipoic acid and pantothenic acid. A deficiency of any of these vitamins could cause malfunctioning of a metabolic pathway at the particular enzymic reaction(s) where the vitamin is involved.

The overall reaction for the oxidation of glucose by living cells is therefore:

$$C_6H_{12}O_6 + 6\,O_2 \longrightarrow 6\,CO_2 + 6\,H_2O + 38\,ATP$$

glucose · oxygen · carbon dioxide · water

The importance of insulin in glucose transport

Insulin is a hormone secreted by the β cells of the pancreas into the blood in response to increased blood glucose concentrations such as might follow a carbohydrate meal. Because of the large mass of muscle and fat tissue in the human body, the ability of insulin to control the uptake and metabolism of glucose in these cells plays a major part in regulating the blood glucose concentration. In diabetes mellitus, where there is inadequate insulin action, the muscle and fat cells are deprived of glucose, and consequently the blood glucose concentration rises (hyperglycaemia). This situation has inspired the aphorism describing diabetes as 'starvation in the midst of plenty'.

If there is an inappropriate excess of insulin relative to the available glucose, then a low blood glucose concentration (hypoglycaemia) results. This might arise if a diabetic patient receives too much insulin in proportion to the carbohydrate supply – or in other words, fails to achieve the balance essential to diabetic control. A rare example of excessive insulin secretion occurs in patients with an insulin-secreting tumour (insulinoma) where the β cells are overactive. In both cases, the resulting hypoglycaemia is dangerous because the brain, which is largely dependent on glucose for fuel, is deprived of its energy supply, and coma may follow.

Insulin is a very important hormone. It has a controlling influence on the metabolism of fats and proteins as well as a direct involvement with glucose metabolism. Its many metabolic actions will be mentioned throughout this book.

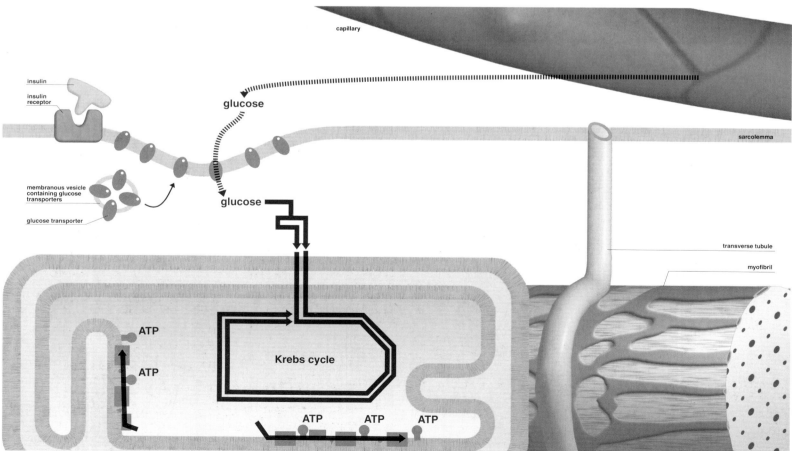

Diagram 5.1. Insulin and the transport of glucose into muscle cells. As shown in Diagram 5.1, glucose is carried by the blood arterial system to the capillaries, which supply the various body tissues. Glucose penetrates the gaps in the capillary wall to form an aqueous fluid, called the interstitial fluid, which bathes the cells. In the case of erythrocytes, liver cells and brain cells, glucose is transported through the outer membrane into the cytosol via a family of insulin-independent facilitative glucose transporters known respectively as Glu T1, Glu T2 and Glu T3. However, in the case of muscle cells (see Diagram, which is not to scale) and fat cells, insulin-dependent glucose transporters are involved. Here, insulin is needed to recruit glucose transporters (of the Glu T4 type) from a latent intracellular location. Insulin causes a vesicle containing the glucose transporters to fuse with the sarcolemma, thereby stimulating glucose transport into the sarcoplasm, where it is oxidized and ATP is formed.

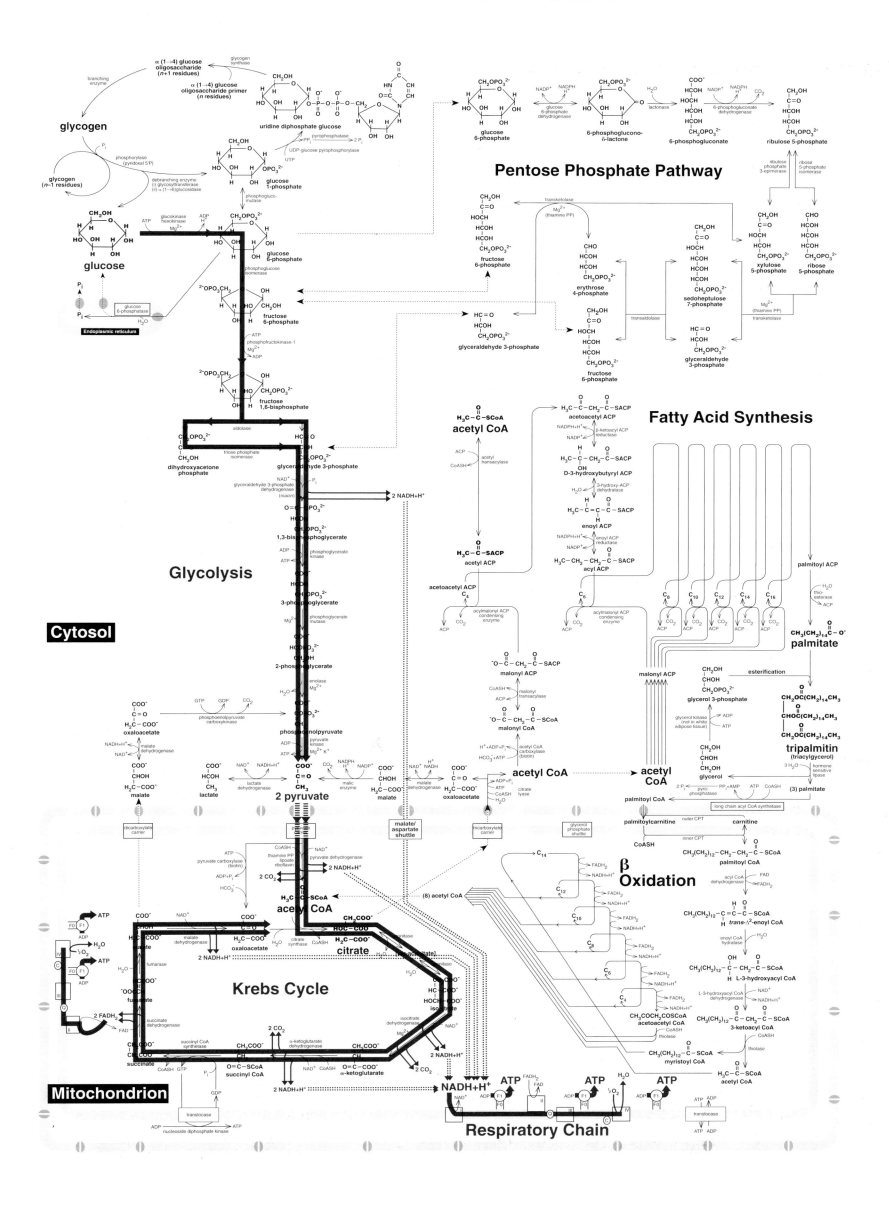

Metabolism of one molecule of glucose to form 38 molecules of ATP

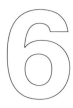

We have considered briefly how living cells oxidize glucose to water and carbon dioxide while the energy is conserved in a biologically useful form as ATP (see Chapter 5). We must now consider the efficiency of ATP production by these metabolic pathways.

Chart 6 opposite. Oxidation of glucose yields 38 molecules of ATP.

Chart 6: Glycolysis

Once glucose has entered the cell it is converted to **glucose 6-phosphate**, a reaction which consumes one molecule of ATP. Glucose 6-phosphate then enters glycolysis and is converted through a series of hexose phosphates to **fructose 1,6-bisphosphate**, requiring yet another ATP molecule to be consumed. Thus, so far, instead of creating ATP, glycolysis has consumed two molecules of this precious energy compound. This initial investment of energy, however, is necessary to activate the substrates and, as we will see, is amply rewarded by a 19-fold net gain.

Fructose 1,6-bisphosphate is then split through the middle into two 3-carbon sugars, namely dihydroxyacetone phosphate and glyceraldehyde 3-phosphate. These two substances are biochemically interconvertible and are frequently referred to collectively as the **triose phosphates**. Because two molecules of triose phosphate are formed, all subsequent reactions are doubled up and are represented in the chart by double lines.

Reduction of glyceraldehyde 3-phosphate and phosphorylation using inorganic phosphate occur to form 1,3-bisphosphoglycerate. This complex oxidation reaction is catalysed by glyceraldehyde 3-phosphate dehydrogenase, and the valuable NADH+H$^+$ formed diffuses through the cytosol, exchanging its hydrogen through the wall of the mitochondrion with assistance from one of the **shuttle systems** (see Chapter 4). In the diagram, for example, the **malate/aspartate** shuttle has been used. The NADH+H$^+$ formed in the mitochondrion then enters the respiratory chain, and three molecules of ATP are formed for each molecule of NADH+H$^+$ oxidized.

Meanwhile, back in the glycolytic pathway, **phosphoglycerate kinase** causes 1,3-bisphosphoglycerate to react with ADP to form 3-phosphoglycerate and ATP. Similarly, three stages further down the pathway, pyruvate kinase causes phosphoenolpyruvate to react with ADP to form pyruvate and ATP.

Krebs cycle

Pyruvate then passes into the mitochondrion and enters the Krebs cycle, where FADH$_2$ and NADH+H$^+$ are formed. FADH$_2$ is the prosthetic group attached to **succinate dehydrogenase**, and donates its electrons via ubiquinone to complex III and thence to complex IV. Accordingly, oxidative phosphorylation of FADH$_2$ produces only two ATP molecules, compared with three from NADH+H$^+$ (see Chapter 2). Also, it should be noted that in the Krebs cycle, GTP is formed by the **succinyl CoA synthetase** reaction. GTP is energetically similar to ATP, to which it is readily converted by **nucleoside diphosphate kinase**.

Overall yield of ATP

From glycolysis	ATP yield
Substrate-level phosphorylation	
Phosphoglycerate kinase	2
Pyruvate kinase	2
Oxidative phosphorylation	
2 NADH+H$^+$ from glyceraldehyde 3-phosphate dehydrogenase	6
	————
	10 ATP

From Krebs cycle	ATP yield
Substrate-level phosphorylation	
Succinyl CoA synthetase (via GTP)	2
Oxidative phosphorylation	
8 NADH+H$^+$	24
2 FADH$_2$	4
	————
	30 ATP

The total gross yield from glycolysis and Krebs cycle is:

10+30=40 molecules of ATP

However, we must not forget that two molecules of ATP were consumed by the glucokinase/hexokinase and phosphofructkinase reactions in the early stages of glycolysis, therefore

the net yield of ATP from glucose =40−2=38 molecules of ATP.

The net yield is 36 ATP molecules in insects

Biochemistry textbooks may appear to contradict each other when describing the yield of ATP from glucose metabolism. Many books show the net energy yield for aerobic glucose metabolism to be 36 ATP molecules, and others quote a yield of 38 molecules, as shown here.

The yield depends on which shuttle system (see Chapter 4) is used to transport cytosolic NADH+H$^+$ into the mitochondrion. In the above calculation it is assumed that the malate/aspartate shuttle is used. However, if the glycerol phosphate shuttle is used, then two NADH+H$^+$ molecules in the cytosol appear as two FADH$_2$ molecules inside the mitochondrion. The final yield of ATP is therefore four from the glycerol phosphate shuttle as opposed to six from the malate/aspartate shuttle. This accounts for the discrepancy referred to above. The glycerol phosphate shuttle is particularly active in insect flight muscle.

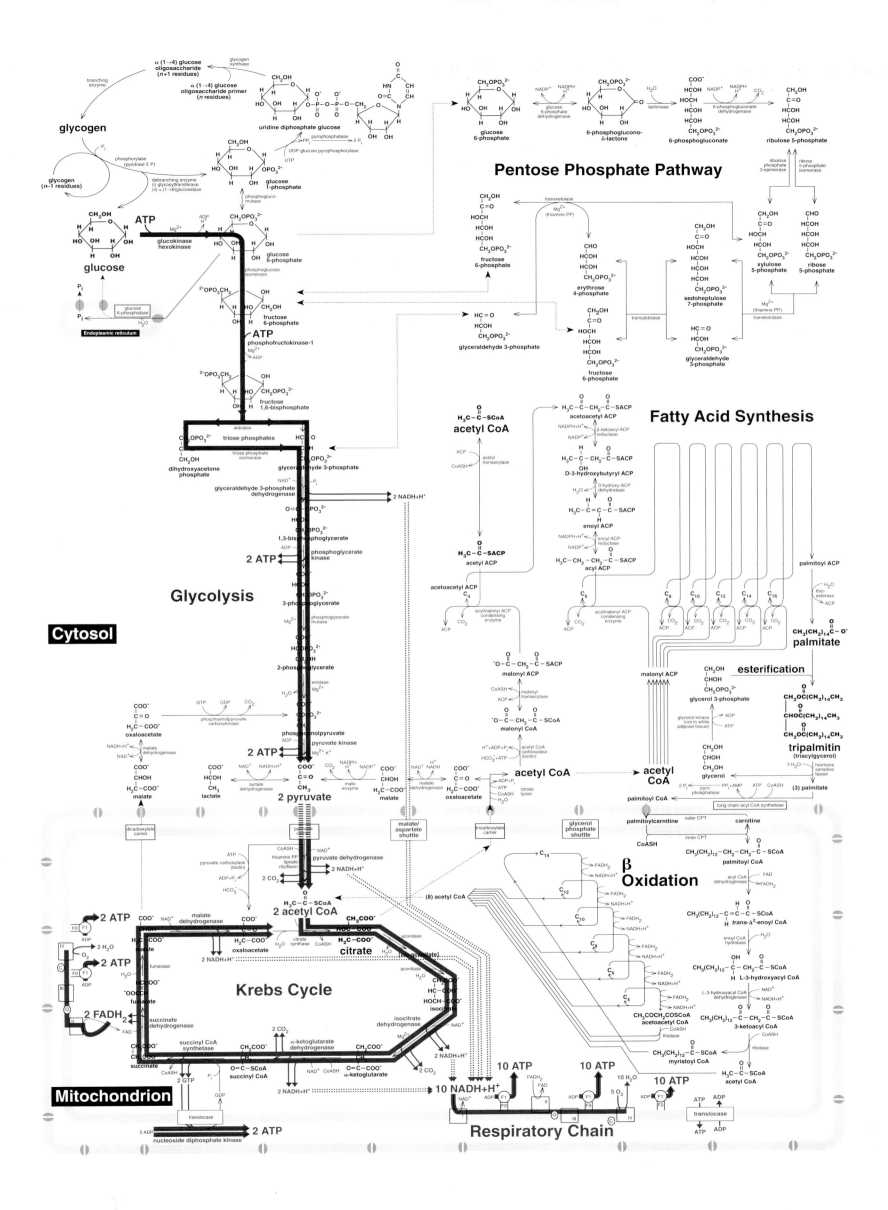

Metabolism of glucose to glycogen

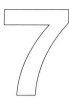

Glycogen is stored in the well-fed state

If we consume large quantities of carbohydrate-rich food in excess of our immediate requirements, then we might expect the concentration of glucose in the blood to rise higher and higher until it eventually assumed the consistency of syrup. If this happened, there would be serious osmotic implications, with water being drawn from the body's cells into the hypertonic blood, causing the former to become dehydrated.

Fortunately, apart from in the diabetic state, this sequence of events does not happen. We have evolved an elaborate control mechanism so that, when provided with a surplus of carbohydrate fuel, it is stored for less bountiful occasions either as **glycogen** or as fat. Glycogen is made from many glucose molecules joined together to form a compact, highly branched, spherical structure.

Chart 7 opposite. Metabolism of glucose to glycogen.

Chart 7: An overview of glycogen synthesis (glycogenesis)

The chart opposite shows how the metabolic fate of glucose can vary according to the energy status of the cell. As we saw in the previous chapter, if the cell needs energy and glucose is available, then the glucose will be oxidized by the glycolytic pathway, the Krebs cycle and the respiratory chain, with the formation of ATP. If, however, the cell is supplied with surplus glucose, causing a high-energy state in the mitochondrion, then the capacity for metabolic flux through the Krebs cycle is overwhelmed and certain metabolites accumulate. Some of these metabolites, such as **citrate**, and **ATP** from the respiratory chain, symbolize an energy surplus and act as messengers (allosteric inhibitors) which inactivate the enzymes of glycolysis. Thus in liver and muscle some of the excess glucose is channelled along the metabolic pathway to glycogen, a process known as **glycogenesis**.

Glycogen as a fuel reserve

The liver and muscles are the major depots for this important energy reserve. The average man who has been well fed on a diet rich in carbohydrate, stores 70 g of glycogen in his liver and 200 g in his muscles. The liver glycogen reserves are sufficient only for an overnight fast at the longest. Accordingly the fat reserves must also be used, especially during long periods of fasting or strenuous exercise.

As we will see later, the brain cannot use fat directly as a fuel and is, to a very great extent, dependent upon a steady supply of glucose via the blood. If the brain is denied glucose it ceases to function properly. The symptoms of a low plasma glucose level include a feeling of dizziness, faintness or lethargy. In hypoglycaemia, defined as a plasma glucose less than 2.5 mmol/l, these symptoms can progress to unconsciousness, coma and, unless glucose is provided rapidly, death.

We can now appreciate the great importance of the reserves of glucose stored as glycogen in the liver. We survive between meals because the liver is able to keep the blood glucose 'topped up' and can maintain a fasting blood concentration of 3.0–5.5 mmol/l, which satisfies the pernickety fuel requirements of the brain.

Glycogen is also an important energy source when confronted with a 'fight or flight' situation. This role will be discussed more fully later (see Chapters 25–28), but as we will see below, the structure of the glycogen molecule is beautifully adapted for the rapid mobilization of glucose in an emergency.

Diagram 7.1: Glycogen, a molecule that is well designed for its function

Glycogen is a complex hydrated polymer of glucose molecules which form a highly branched spherical structure. The very large molecular weight, which ranges over several million daltons, enables glucose to be stored without the osmotic complications associated with free glucose molecules. The size of the glycogen molecule varies with the prevailing nutritional status, being larger (up to 40 nm in diameter) in the well-fed state, and progressively shrinking to around 10 nm or less between meals.

The glucose chain is attached to the protein **glycogenin**. The glucose molecules are joined by $\alpha(1\rightarrow4)$ glycosidic bonds, except at the branch points, which are $\alpha(1\rightarrow6)$ glycosidic bonds. A branch occurs, on average, every 10 glucose units along the chain. This highly branched spherical structure creates a large number of exposed terminal glucose molecules, which are accessible to the enzymes involved in glycogen breakdown (glycogenolysis). This ensures an extremely rapid release of glucose units from glycogen in the 'fight or flight' emergency situation, which can sometimes be vital for survival.

Diagram 7.1. Diagrammatic representation of a glycogen molecule.

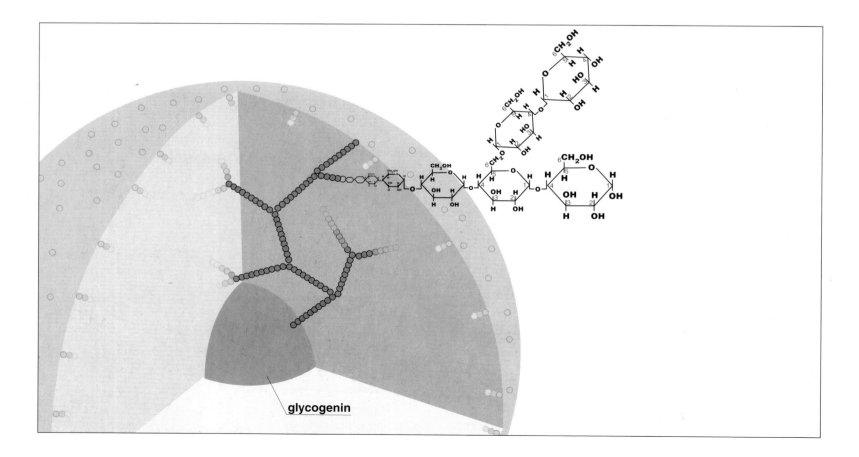

glycogenin

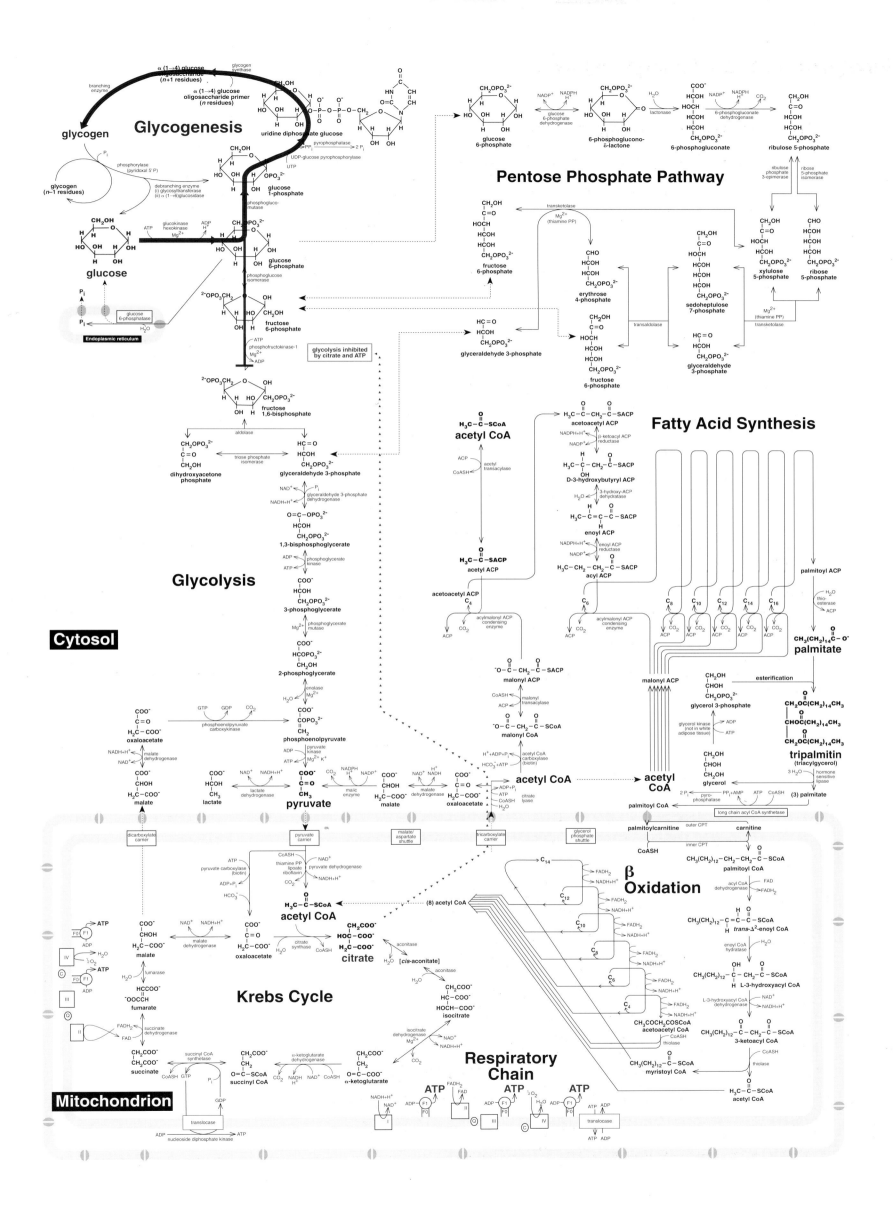

Anaerobic metabolism of glucose and glycogen to yield energy as ATP

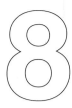

Chart 8 opposite. Anaerobic metabolism of glucose and glycogen to yield energy as ATP.

Anaerobic glycolysis

We have already seen how, in the presence of oxygen, glucose and glycogen are oxidized to carbon dioxide and water, with energy being conserved as ATP (see Chapter 6). However, glucose and glycogen can also be oxidized **anaerobically**: that is, without oxygen. This process is particularly important in exercising muscle. It enables muscle to generate ATP very rapidly and at a rate faster than would be permitted by the availability of oxygen from the air. In practice, this means that eventually we become 'out of breath' and then have to rest to repay the 'oxygen debt'.

Anaerobic glycolysis is also very important in the retina, kidney medulla and, paradoxically, in red blood cells in spite of the abundance of oxygen in the latter, see below.

Chart 8: Glucose is metabolized to lactate

Anaerobic oxidation proceeds as shown in the chart. **Glucose** and **glycogen** are metabolized by glycolysis to **pyruvate** and four ATP molecules are produced. However, NAD^+ is reduced to $NADH+H^+$ by **glyceraldehyde 3-phosphate dehydrogenase**. Normally, in the presence of oxygen, this $NADH+H^+$ equivalent (see Chapter 4) would enter the mitochondria and be oxidized to regenerate NAD^+. Since glycolysis needs a constant supply of NAD^+, the problem is, how is NAD^+ regenerated without oxygen?

The enzyme **lactate dehydrogenase** provides the answer. This enzyme catalyses the reduction of pyruvate to **lactate**, and simultaneously NADH is oxidized to NAD^+. The regenerated NAD^+ is thus free to serve glyceraldehyde 3-phosphate dehydrogenase as a coenzyme. In this way, glycolysis continues but lactate accumulates. This represents the 'oxygen debt' which must be repaid, when oxygen is available, by oxidizing the accumulated lactate to pyruvate in the liver. The pyruvate so formed can then be converted to glucose.

ATP yield by anaerobic metabolism

Anaerobic glycolysis from glucose

Molecules of ATP formed	4
Less 2 ATP to activate glycolysis	–2
Net ATP total	2

Anaerobic glycolysis from glycogen

Molecules of ATP formed	4
Less 1 ATP to initiate glycolysis	–1
Net ATP total	3

The above anaerobic pathways, which produce a net yield of two and three ATP molecules respectively, are very inefficient compared with the net yield from aerobic pathways, namely 38 molecules of ATP (see Chapter 6). Nevertheless, the ability to generate ATP rapidly in the absence of oxygen is vital to the survival of many species.

Physiological and clinical relevance
Anaerobic glycolysis for 'fuel-injection' performance

Adrenaline, as part of the 'fight or flight' response, stimulates the breakdown of glycogen and thus glycolysis. This pathway is especially important in fast-twitch (white) muscle, which is relatively deficient in oxidative metabolism due to a poor blood supply and few mitochondria. White muscle is found, for example, in the flight muscles of some game birds, e.g. grouse. It is well adapted for an explosive burst of energy, thus helping these animals to evade predators.

When oxygen becomes more plentiful again, the rate of glycolysis falls dramatically as more efficient oxidation involving the Krebs cycle is activated. This adaptation is known as the 'Pasteur effect' after Louis Pasteur, who first observed this phenomenon in yeast (see Chapter 29).

Hyperlactataemia and lactic acidosis

The blood concentration of lactate is normally around 1 mmol/l. Since the pK of lactic acid is 3.86, it is completely dissociated to form lactate anions and hydrogen ions at normal blood pH. If the concentration of lactate is increased up to 5 mmol/l, this is known as hyperlactataemia. If it exceeds 5 mmol/l, and the bicarbonate buffer system is overwhelmed, the condition is described as lactic acidosis and the blood pH may decrease from the normal range of 7.35–7.45 to around pH 7 or below. Lactic acidosis may result from increased lactate production due to tissue hypoxia. Alternatively, it may also result from decreased removal of lactate by the liver for gluconeogenesis due to disease or a reduced hepatic blood supply.

Lactic acidosis and disease

Lactic acidosis is often due to the generalized tissue hypoxia associated with shock or congestive cardiac failure. Here, two factors contribute to lactate accumulation. These are an inadequate oxygen supply to the tissue, causing increased anaerobic glycolysis with increased lactate production; and a decreased clearance of lactate from the blood.

A mild hyperlactataemia may also occur in thiamine deficiency. This is because **pyruvate dehydrogenase** needs **thiamine** for activity and, consequently, removal of pyruvate is obstructed. Since lactate dehydrogenase activity is high in cells, it maintains pyruvate and lactate at equilibrium, so that when pyruvate accumulates so also does lactate.

Diagram 8.1: The Cori cycle

If our muscles need energy in an emergency or for a sprint racing event such as a 200 m race, then most of the ATP used will be derived from anaerobic breakdown of muscle glycogen by glycolysis. The diagram shows that lactate formed during this process diffuses from the muscle into the capillaries, and is transported to the liver, entering the lobules via the hepatic arterioles. Then, provided the liver cells are adequately oxygenated, the lactate is oxidized to pyruvate which may be reconverted to glucose by the process known as gluconeogenesis (see Chapter 31). The glucose so formed may be exported from the liver via the central vein and thus made available again to the muscle for energy purposes or for storage as glycogen. This is known as 'the Cori cycle'.

Red blood cells

Mature red blood cells do not contain mitochondria and are therefore exclusively dependent on anaerobic oxidation of glucose for their ATP supply. The lactate produced diffuses from the red cell into the plasma and thence to the liver, where it is oxidized to pyruvate and may then be reconverted to glucose (the Cori cycle). In laboratory medicine, fluoride is used as a preservative for blood glucose samples from diabetic patients because it inhibits the glycolytic enzyme **enolase**, which converts 2-phosphoglycerate to phosphoenolpyruvate.

Diagram 8.1. The Cori cycle.

glycogen

glucose

glycolysis

Muscle

lactate ← pyruvate

Liver

glucose ←

gluconeogenesis

lactate → pyruvate

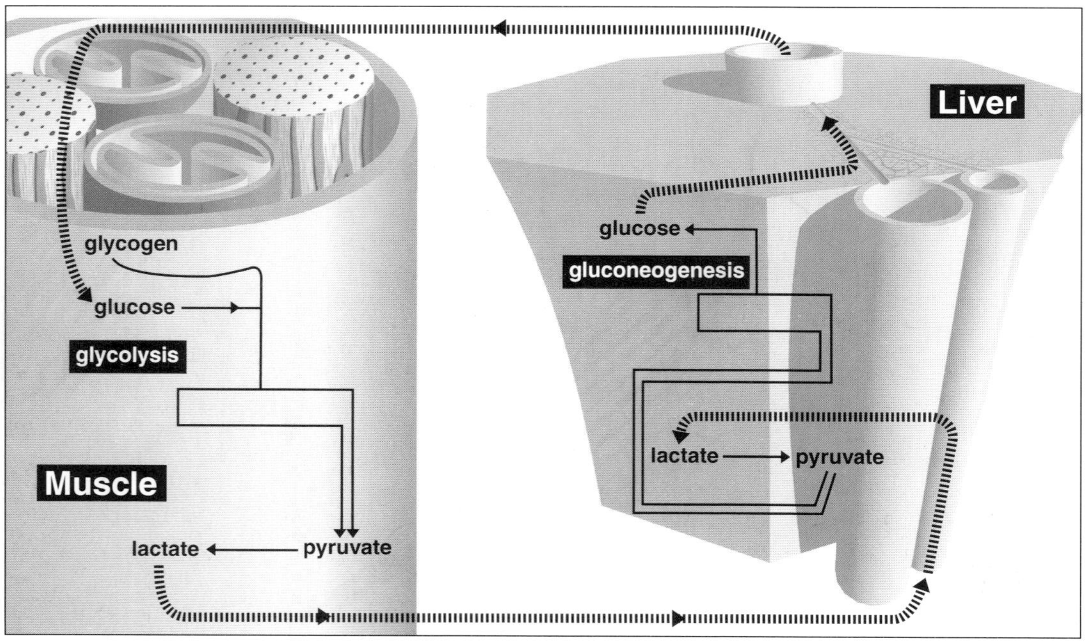

2,3-Bisphosphoglycerate (2,3-BPG) and the red blood cell

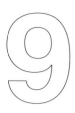

Chart 9 opposite. 2,3-BPG metabolism.

2,3-BPG helps to unload oxygen from haemoglobin

Haemoglobin, the oxygen-carrying protein found in red blood cells, has a high binding affinity for oxygen and can therefore transport oxygen to the tissues where it is needed. The problem then is that, on arrival at the tissues, haemoglobin must be persuaded to release its tightly bound cargo. It has been known since the early 1900s that the presence of H^+ ions in contracting muscle unloads oxygen from the haemoglobin. This is known as the 'Bohr effect'. However, it has been known only since 1967 that there is another factor, **2,3-BPG** (2,3-bisphosphoglycerate, called 2,3-DPG (2,3-diphosphoglycerate) in medical circles), which is an allosteric effector that binds to deoxyhaemoglobin, thereby lowering its affinity for oxygen.

Whereas the response to H^+ ions is very rapid, 2,3-BPG operates over longer periods, allowing adaptations to gradual changes in oxygen availability.

Chart 9: The 2,3-BPG shunt in red blood cells (Rapoport–Luebering shunt)

The chart shows only glycolysis and the pentose phosphate pathway, since the other pathways shown in previous and subsequent chapters are not present in mature red blood cells.

The shunt consists of **bisphosphoglycerate mutase** and **2,3-bisphosphate phosphatase**. Bisphosphoglycerate mutase is stimulated by 3-phosphoglycerate, which causes increased production of 2,3-BPG. **NB:** When this shunt operates, ATP is not produced by the phosphoglycerate kinase reaction. This means that ATP is produced exclusively by the pyruvate kinase reaction, but there is no net gain of ATP from glycolysis under these circumstances.

Physiological significance of 2,3-BPG
Fetal haemoglobin has a low affinity for 2,3-BPG

Fetal haemoglobin is a tetramer of two α chains and two γ chains, unlike adult haemoglobin which comprises two α and two β chains. Fetal haemoglobin has a lower affinity for 2,3-BPG than adult haemoglobin, and consequently it has a higher affinity for oxygen. This facilitates placental exchange of oxygen from the mother to the fetus.

2,3-BPG and adaptation to high altitude

Anyone accustomed to living at low altitude who has flown to a high-altitude location will be aware that even moderate exertion will cause breathlessness. Within a few days, adaptation occurs as the concentration of 2,3-BPG in red cells increases, enabling the tissues to obtain oxygen in spite of its relatively diminished availability in the thin mountain air. On returning to low altitude the concentration of 2,3-BPG, which has a half-life of 6 hours, returns rapidly to normal.

Importance of 2,3-BPG in medicine
Blood transfusions

Haematologists have long known that blood which has been stored prior to transfusion has an unusually high affinity for oxygen. This is because 2,3-BPG, which forms 65% of the organic phosphates of red cells, disappears on storing in acid-citrate–glucose medium, the concentration falling from about 5 mmol/l to 0.5 mmol/l in 10 days. Consequently, in theory, it would be expected that if a patient is given a large volume of stored blood, the red cells would be unable to unload their oxygen and so, in spite of the presence of oxygen, tissue hypoxia would result. However, in modern clinical practice this is prevented by using anticoagulants and additives (e.g. saline, adenine, glucose, mannitol), which minimize depletion of 2,3-BPG.

Deficiency of red-cell glycolytic enzymes

Patients with inherited diseases due to deficiencies of red-cell glycolytic enzymes are unable to transport oxygen normally. However, the nature of the effect on 2,3-BPG concentrations depends on whether the deficiency is proximal or distal to the 2,3-BPG shunt. In patients with proximal deficiencies, e.g. **hexokinase**, **phosphoglucose isomerase**, **phosphofructokinase** and **aldolase** deficiencies, there is a reduced flow of metabolites through glycolysis, and consequently the 2,3-BPG concentration falls. There is therefore an associated tendency towards tissue hypoxia, since the haemoglobin maintains its high affinity for oxygen. In enzymopathies distal to the shunt, e.g. **pyruvate kinase** deficiency, the opposite situation prevails. Here, the glycolytic intermediates accumulate and, as a result, the concentration of 2,3-BPG is about twice normal. This means that in this condition haemoglobin has a relatively low affinity for, and ability to transport, oxygen.

Finally, patients have been reported with deficiency of the shunt enzymes, **BPG mutase** and **2,3-BPG phosphatase**, suggesting that both activities reside in the same protein. As would be expected, concentrations of 2,3-BPG are severely decreased in these patients, who have an increase in red-cell mass to compensate for the diminished supply of oxygen to the tissues.

Hypophosphataemia during therapy for diabetic ketoacidosis

This may result from intravenous infusion of glucose postoperatively, or may occur after insulin treatment for diabetic ketoacidosis. This is because of the acute demand for phosphate by the tissues to form the phosphorylated intermediates of metabolism. Unfortunately, the fall in plasma phosphate causes low concentrations of phosphate in red cells. This results in decreased 2,3-BPG levels, which in turn causes tissue hypoxia.

It has been suggested that, during glucose infusion and during treatment for diabetic ketoacidosis, phosphate replacement might minimize tissue hypoxia and so assist recovery. However, clinical studies have shown that, whereas phosphate therapy might accelerate the regeneration of 2,3-BPG in red cells, there were no demonstrable clinical benefits to the patients.

Common causes of increased red-cell 2,3-BPG concentrations

The concentration of 2,3-BPG is increased in smokers, which compensates for a diminished oxygen supply because of their chronic exposure to carbon monoxide. Also, a compensatory increase in 2,3-BPG is commonly found in patients with chronic anaemia.

Myoglobin

Myoglobin is very similar to the β chain of haemoglobin and it also has a high affinity for oxygen. Although 2,3-BPG has no direct effect on myoglobin, this important protein and its role in oxygen transport must not be overlooked. It provides a reserve supply of oxygen and, as such, is particularly abundant in the skeletal muscle of aquatic mammals such as whales and seals, enabling them to remain submerged for several minutes.

Diagram 9.1: Transport of oxygen from the red blood cell to the mitochondrion for use in oxidative phosphorylation

This shows the route by which oxygen is transported from haemoglobin to the mitochondrion. First, oxygen is dissociated from haemoglobin in red cells and diffuses through the capillary wall into the extracellular fluid, and on into the muscle cell. Here, oxygen is bound to myoglobin until required by complex IV of the respiratory chain for oxidative phosphorylation.

Reference

Fisher J. N. and Kitabchi A. E., A randomised study of phosphate therapy in the treatment of diabetic ketoacidosis. *J Clin Endocrinol Metab* **57**, 177–180, 1983.

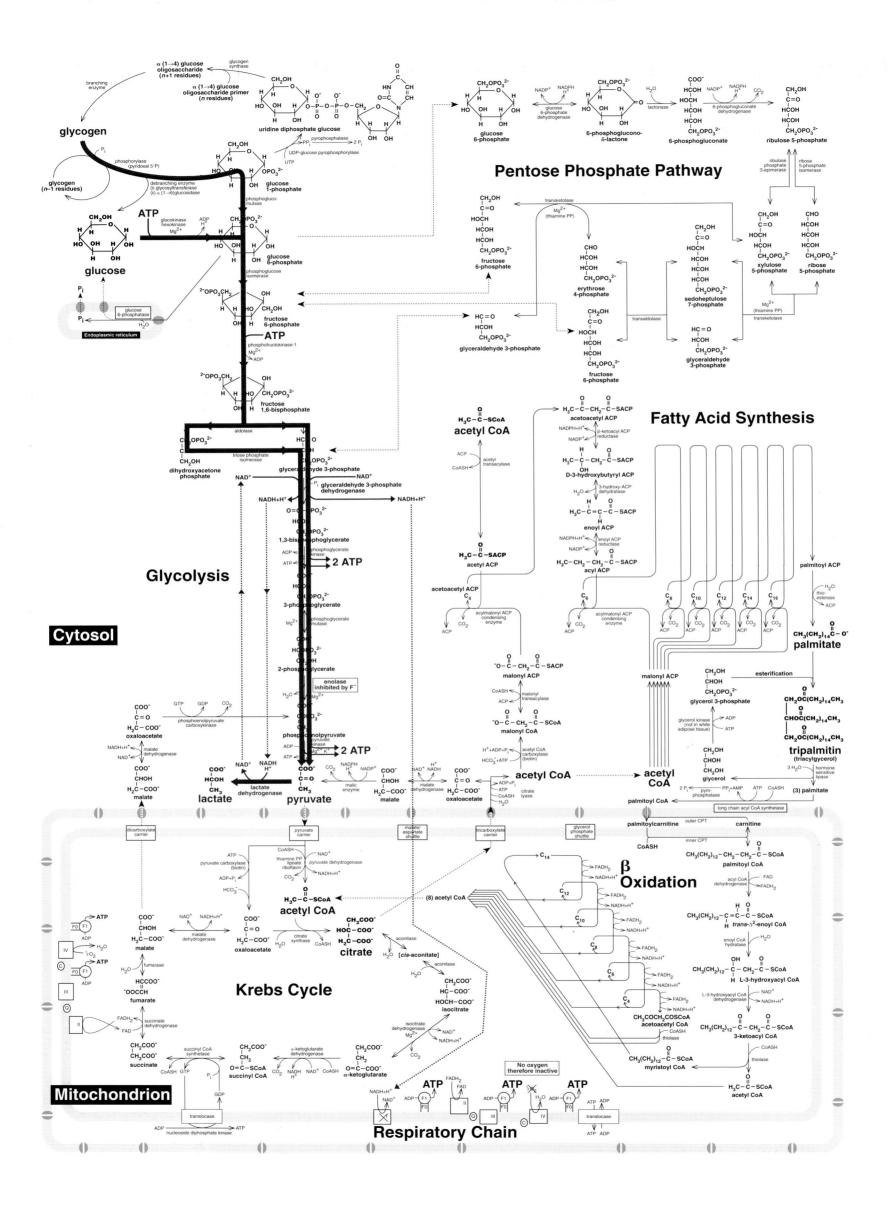

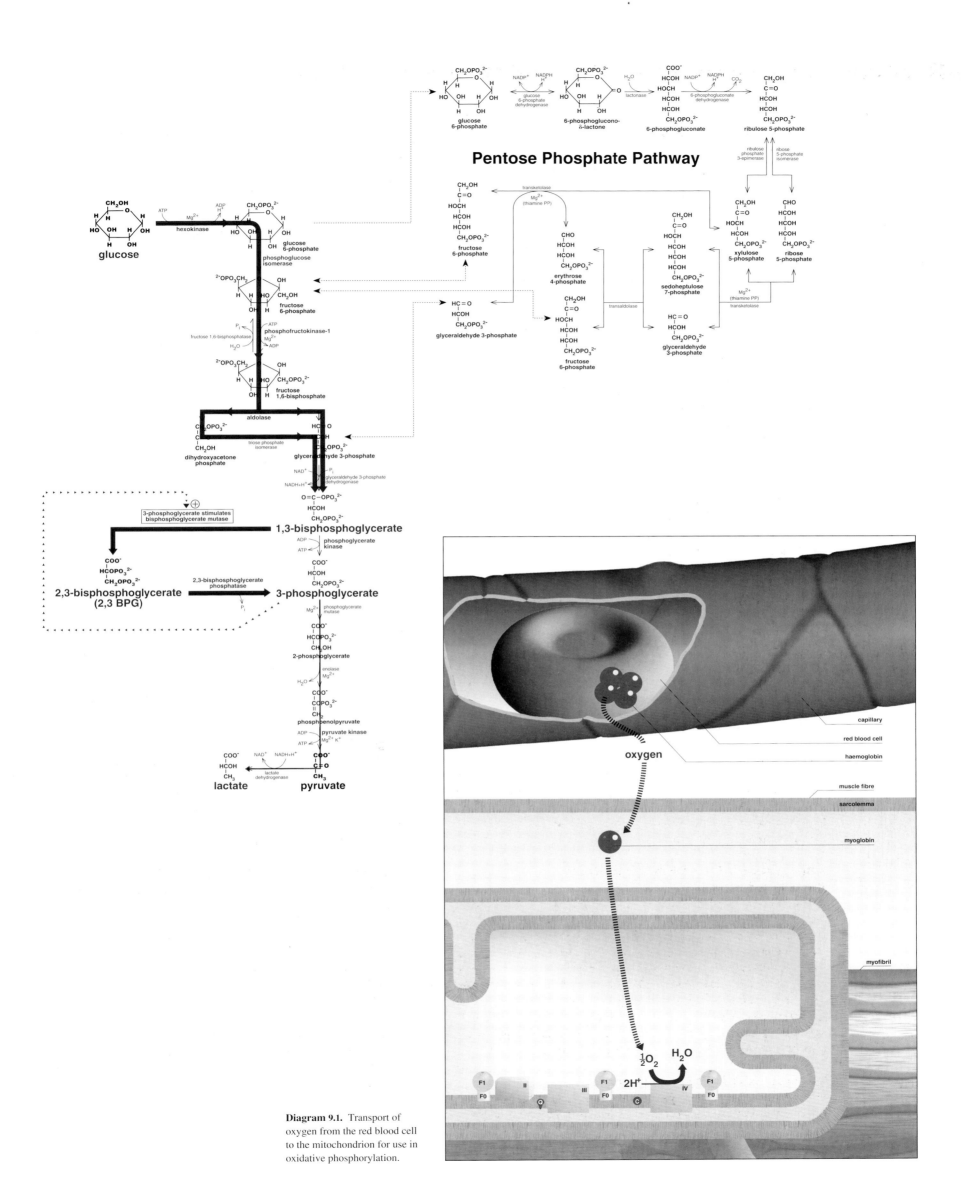

Diagram 9.1. Transport of oxygen from the red blood cell to the mitochondrion for use in oxidative phosphorylation.

Metabolism of glucose to fat (triacylglycerol)

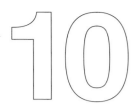

10

Chart 10 opposite. Metabolism of glucose to triacylglycerol.

The importance of fat

The statement 'if you eat too much food, you will become fat' is unlikely to surprise any reader of this book. We know from experience that a surplus of fat in our diet will increase the fat in our body. Furthermore, it is general knowledge that an excess of carbohydrate will be stored as fat. However, a surprising number of people enjoy life under the delusion that they can eat large amounts of protein without the hazard of becoming fat. Sadly, this misconception will be shattered by reality in Chapter 21. Let us turn to the physiological advantages of body fat. Primitive man, like many other carnivorous mammals that hunted for food, was an intermittent feeder. In the days before refrigeration he was unable to store joints from his woolly mammoth in the deep-freeze, to be divided subsequently into a gastronomical routine of breakfast, lunch, dinner and supper. Instead, when food was available the hunters and their families ate all they could, with any surplus to immediate energy requirements being stored in the body, to a certain extent as glycogen but mainly as fat. This fat can provide an energy store for sustenance over periods of starvation lasting several days or even weeks.

Fat provides a very compact store for energy, largely because of its highly reduced and anhydrous nature. In fact, 1 g of fat yields 9 kcal (37 kJ). This compares well with 1 g of carbohydrate: 3.75 kcal (16 kJ); or protein: 4 kcal (17 kJ).

Liver cells and fat cells (adipocytes) are both major producers of fat. In addition, with the onset of lactation at the end of pregnancy, the mammary gland develops almost overnight the ability to synthesize prodigious amounts of fat for secretion in the milk.

Chart 10: The flow of metabolites when glucose is converted to triacylglycerol

The chart shows the metabolic pathways involved when a surplus of carbohydrate is taken in the diet. We have seen how the liver is able to conserve useful, but limited, supplies of energy as glycogen (see Chapter 7). Once these glycogen reserves are full, any additional carbohydrate will be converted to fat as follows: glucose enters the pentose phosphate pathway, the metabolites of which form a temporary diversion from the glycolytic pathway. The metabolites eventually rejoin the main glycolytic route, pass into the mitochondrion and enter the Krebs cycle. However, in the well-fed state the mitochondrial pathways will be working to capacity and generating large amounts of ATP and NADH+H$^+$. Under these circumstances, a control mechanism (see Chapter 30) diverts citrate from the Krebs cycle into the cytosol for fatty acid synthesis (see Chapter 11). Although Chart 10 shows the formation of **palmitate**, stearate is also formed by this pathway. Both can be esterified and incorporated into **triacylglycerols**. **NB:** The vitamin **biotin** is an essential cofactor for the regulatory enzyme **acetyl CoA carboxylase** in the pathway for fatty acid synthesis.

Diagram 10.1: Insulin and fat synthesis

Adipocytes are the specialized cells of adipose tissue where triacylglycerols are synthesized and stored. They contain the usual cellular organelles but, because the cell interior is almost completely occupied by a large, spherical fat droplet, the cytosol and organelles are displaced to the periphery. Adipose tissue is widely distributed, being found beneath the skin and especially around the intestines, kidneys and other visceral organs.

Blood capillaries in adipose tissue bring supplies of glucose for fatty acid synthesis. The diagram shows the relationship between adipocytes and a capillary, but is not to scale: in reality, the adipocytes would be much larger. The glucose passes through the capillary wall into the extracellular fluid. After feeding, insulin is released from the pancreas and causes 30-fold increased rate of transport of glucose into the adipocyte. Insulin causes the translocation of a latent pool of Glu T4, glucose transporters from within the adipocyte cytosol to the plasma membrane. These facilitate the transport of glucose into the cytosol, where it is metabolized to triacylglycerols, which are stored as a spherical droplet as described earlier.

Not all the body's triacylglycerol is made by the adipose tissue. Triacylglycerol is usually available in food and is absorbed from the gut as chylomicrons, whose role is to transport the triacylglycerols from the intestines to the adipocytes for storage. Alternatively, the liver makes triacylglycerols for export in a protein–phospholipid-coated package known as a VLDL (very low-density lipoprotein). Similarly, these VLDLs transport triacylglycerol to adipose tissue for storage.

Diagram 10.1. Insulin stimulates the transport of glucose into adipocytes for triacylglycerol synthesis.

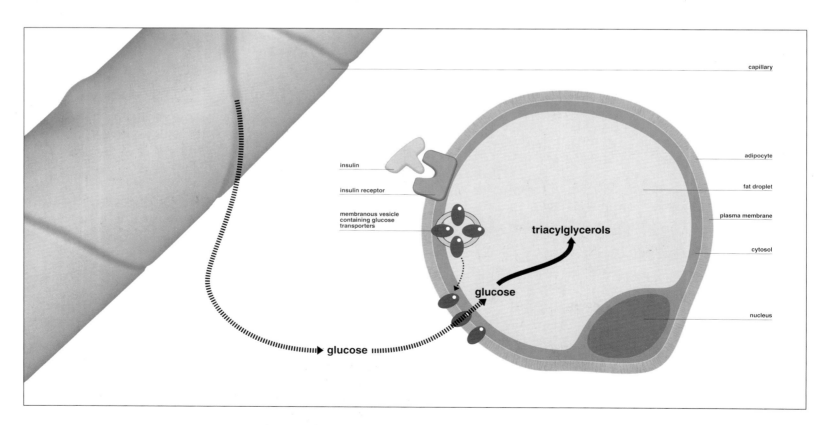

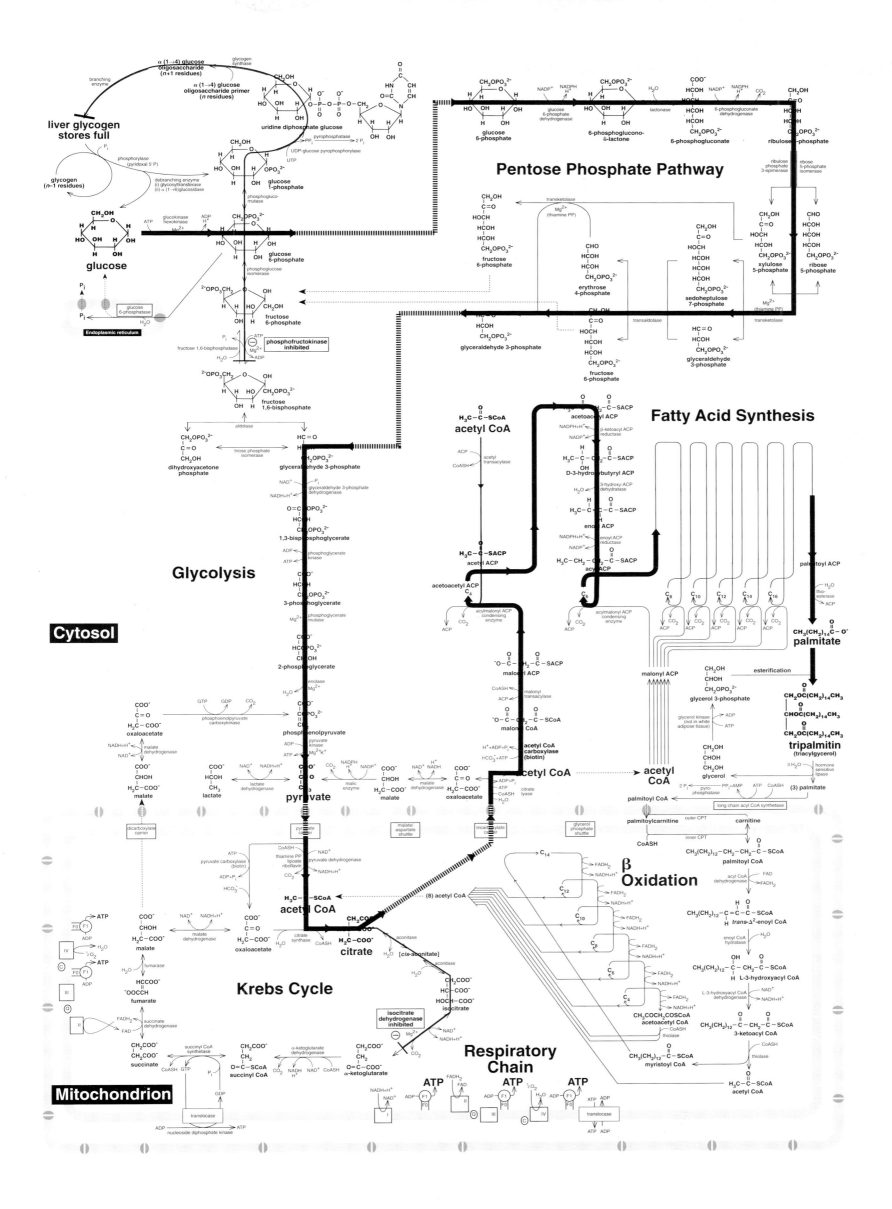

Metabolism of glucose to fatty acids and triacylglycerol

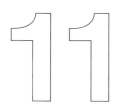

A brief description of how glucose is converted to fat appeared in Chapter 10. It is now time to look at triacylglycerol biosynthesis in more detail.

The liver, adipose tissue and lactating mammary gland are the principal tissues involved in lipogenesis (triacylglycerol synthesis). Liver and adipose tissue make triacylglycerol from glucose under conditions of abundant carbohydrate intake; in other words, when the body has more than enough food to satisfy its immediate needs for energy.

Chart 11 opposite. Metabolism of fatty acids and triacylglycerol.

Chart 11: Synthesis of triacylglycerols from glucose
The importance of citrate in activating fatty acid synthesis
The mitochondrion in the high-energy state has large quantities of ATP and NADH+H⁺. These metabolites, both symbols of cellular affluence, reduce the rate of flow of metabolites through the Krebs cycle by inhibiting **isocitrate dehydrogenase**. Consequently, the metabolites isocitrate and **citrate** accumulate, and their concentration within the mitochondrion increases. As the concentration of citrate rises, it diffuses via the **tricarboxylate carrier** from the mitochondrion into the cytosol, where citrate serves three functions:

1 Citrate, and ATP, are allosteric regulators that reduce the metabolic flux through glycolysis by inhibiting **phosphofructokinase-1**, thereby redirecting metabolites into the pentose phosphate pathway. This pathway produces NADPH+H⁺, which is an essential coenzyme for fatty acid synthesis.
2 Citrate in the cytosol is split by **citrate lyase** (the citrate cleavage enzyme) to form **oxaloacetate** and **acetyl CoA**. The latter is the precursor for fatty acid synthesis.
3 Citrate activates **acetyl CoA carboxylase**, which is a regulatory enzyme controlling fatty acid synthesis.

In these three ways, citrate has organized the metabolic pathways of the liver or fat cell so that lipogenesis may proceed.

The pentose phosphate pathway generates NADPH+H⁺ for fatty acid synthesis
To reiterate, once the immediate energy demands of the animal have been satisfied, surplus glucose will be stored in the liver as glycogen. When the glycogen stores are full, any surplus glucose molecules will find the glycolytic pathway inhibited at the level of phosphofructokinase. Under these circumstances, the metabolic flux via the pentose phosphate pathway is

stimulated. This is a complex pathway generating **glyceraldehyde 3-phosphate**, which then re-enters glycolysis, thus bypassing the inhibition at phosphofructokinase. Because of this bypass, the pathway is sometimes referred to as the 'hexose monophosphate shunt' pathway.

One very important feature of the pentose phosphate pathway is that it produces **NADPH+H⁺** from **NADP⁺**. NADPH+H⁺ is a hydrogen carrier which is derived from the vitamin niacin, and as such is a phosphorylated form of NAD⁺, the important functional difference being that, whereas NADH+H⁺ is used for ATP production, NADPH+H⁺ is used for fatty acid synthesis and other biosynthetic reactions.

Fatty acid synthesis and esterification
Starting from glucose, the chart shows the metabolic flux via the pentose phosphate pathway and glycolysis to mitochondrial acetyl CoA, and hence via citrate to acetyl CoA in the cytosol. Fatty acid synthesis is catalysed by the fatty acid synthase complex which requires malonyl CoA. The latter combines with the **acyl carrier protein (ACP)** to form **malonyl ACP**. Fatty acid synthesis proceeds via the cyclical series of of reactions as shown in the chart to form **palmitate** (and also stearate, which is not shown). However, fat is stored not as fatty acids but as **triacylglycerols** (triglycerides). These are made by a series of esterification reactions which combine three fatty acid molecules with **glycerol 3-phosphate** (see Chapter 32).

Diagram 11.1: Activation of acetyl CoA carboxylase by citrate *in vitro*
Experiments *in vitro* have shown that acetyl CoA carboxylase exists as units (or protomers), which are enzymically inactive. However, citrate causes these protomers to polymerize and form enzymically active filaments which promote fatty acid synthesis. Conversely, the product of the reaction, namely fatty acyl CoA (palmitoyl CoA), causes depolymerization of the filament. Kinetic studies have shown that, whereas polymerization is very rapid, taking only a few seconds, depolymerization is much slower, with a half-life of approximately 10 minutes. The length of a polymer varies, but on average consists of 20 units, and it has been calculated that a single liver cell contains 50000 such filaments.

Each of the units contains biotin and is a dimer of two identical polypeptide subunits. The activity is also regulated by hormonally mediated phosphorylation/dephosphorylation reactions (see Chapter 32).

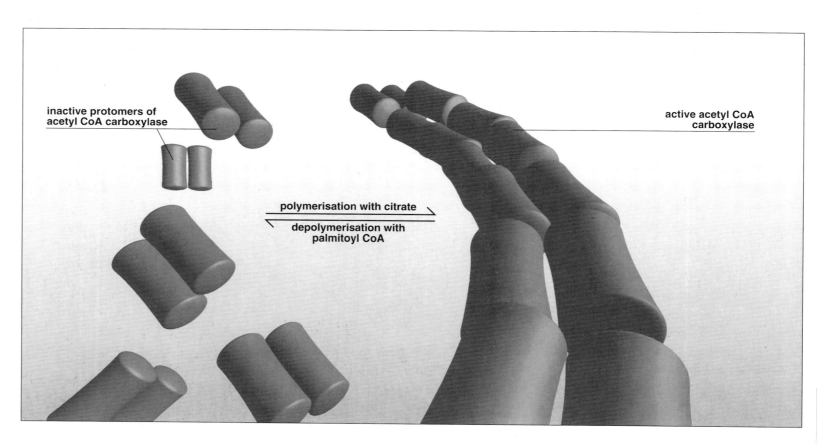

inactive protomers of acetyl CoA carboxylase

active acetyl CoA carboxylase

polymerisation with citrate

depolymerisation with palmitoyl CoA

Diagram 11.1. Activation of acetyl CoA carboxylase by citrate.

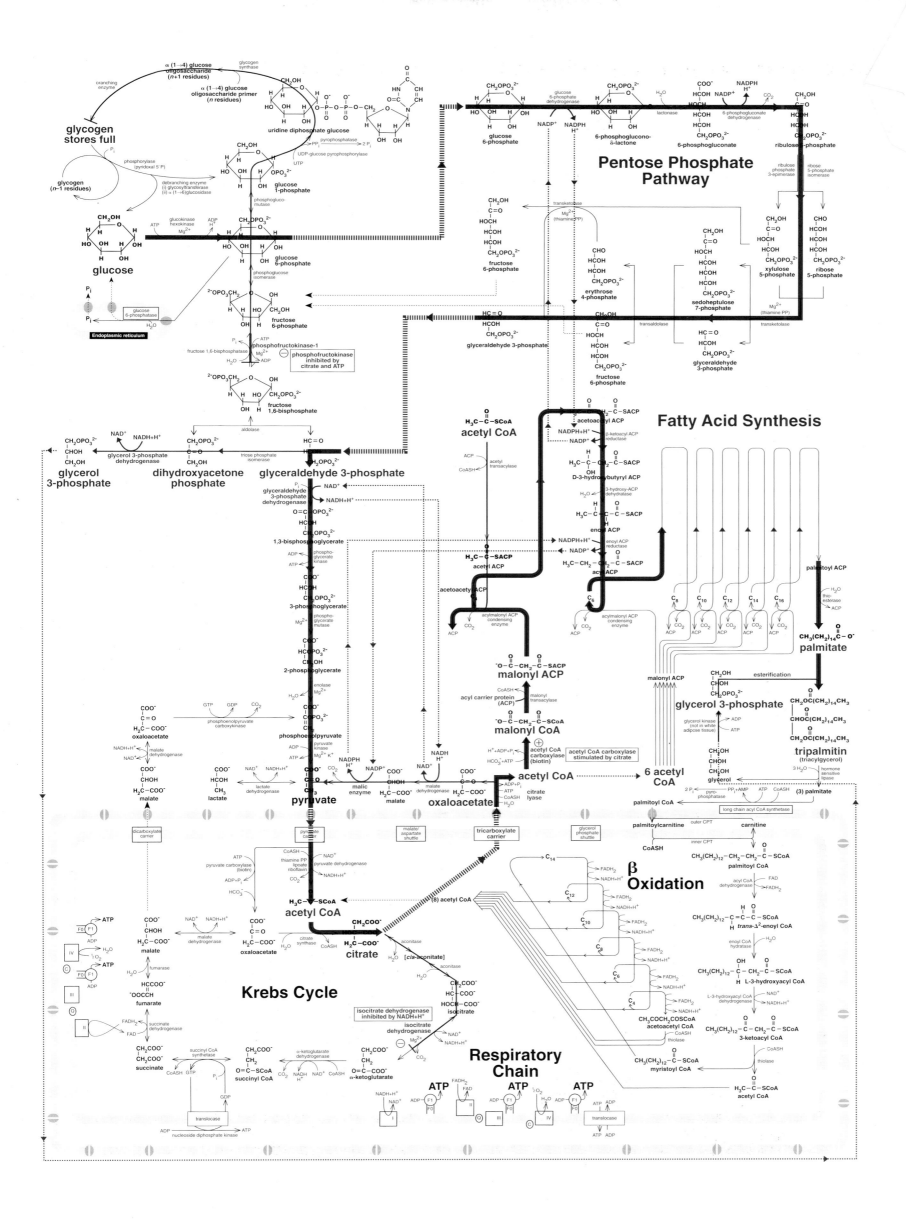

12

Chart 12 opposite. The pentose phosphate pathway provides NADPH+H$^+$ for lipogenesis.

The pentose phosphate pathway

In mammals, the pentose phosphate pathway (also known as the hexose monophosphate shunt or the phosphogluconate pathway) is active only in liver, adipose tissue, lactating mammary gland, adrenal cortex and red blood cells. In these tissues it provides 'reducing power' in the form of NADPH+H$^+$. This NADPH+H$^+$ is used for the biosynthesis of fatty acids and cholesterol and, particularly in red blood cells, the production of glutathione. In plants, the pathway is involved in the photosynthetic dark reaction.

Another important function is to produce ribose 5-phosphate for nucleotide and nucleic acid synthesis. However, as described later, only the 'reversible, non-oxidative phase' of the pathway, which is ubiquitous, is needed for this process.

Chart 12: The pentose phosphate pathway

The pathway can be considered in two phases: the 'irreversible oxidative phase' comprising the reactions catalysed by glucose 6-phosphate dehydrogenase, lactonase and 6-phosphogluconate dehydrogenase; and the 'reversible, non-oxidative phase' involving the rest of the pathway.

Irreversible, oxidative phase of the pentose phosphate pathway

The stoichiometry of the pentose phosphate pathway can be studied by following the metabolic fate of three molecules of glucose. In the well-fed state, glucose is phosphorylated to glucose 6-phosphate. Remember that phosphofructokinase is inhibited by the abundance of ATP and citrate in the high-energy state. Accordingly glucose 6-phosphate enters the pentose phosphate pathway, where it is oxidized by glucose 6-phosphate dehydrogenase and NADPH+H$^+$ is formed. Also produced is 6-phosphoglucono-δ-lactone, which is rapidly and irreversibly hydrolysed by lactonase. Next, 6-phosphogluconate dehydrogenase irreversibly produces ribulose 5-phosphate, another molecule of NADPH+H$^+$, and CO$_2$ is evolved. Henceforth, the flux of metabolites is committed to the next phase of the pathway.

Reversible, non-oxidative phase of the pentose phosphate pathway

This involves reactions that convert three molecules of **ribulose 5-phosphate** to two molecules of fructose 6-phosphate and one molecule of glyceraldehyde 3-phosphate. **NB:** ribose 5-phosphate is a precursor of nucleotide synthesis.

The fate of fructose 6-phosphate

Fructose 6-phosphate could now be converted back to glucose 6-phosphate by the equilibrium reaction catalysed by **phosphoglucose isomerase** for re-entry into the pentose phosphate pathway in a cyclical manner (Diagram 12.2). This cycle is important in red blood cells, where the NADPH+H$^+$ produced is used to synthesize **reduced glutathione**.

However, the fate of fructose 6-phosphate is as indicated in Chart 12, in liver and adipose tissue where lipogenesis prevails in the well-fed state. When dietary carbohydrate is absorbed by the intestines, a surge of glucose is delivered to the liver and adipose tissue and a high concentration of glucose 6-phosphate is produced. This favours fructose 6-phosphate formation, which accumulates until its concentration is sufficient to overcome the ATP-induced inhibition of phosphofructokinase (Diagram 12.1). Two molecules of fructose 6-phosphate produce two molecules of fructose 1,6-bisphosphate which, following cleavage by aldolase and the triose phosphate isomerase reaction, yield four molecules of glyceraldehyde 3-phosphate. Including the glyceraldehyde 3-phosphate formed in the pentose phosphate pathway, a total of five glyceraldehyde 3-phosphate molecules continue through glycolysis to form five molecules of pyruvate, which, in the lipogenic state, can enter the pyruvate/malate cycle (see Chapter 13).

Regulation of the pentose phosphate pathway

The flow of metabolites through the pathway is regulated at the glucose 6-phosphate dehydrogenase reaction and the 6-phosphogluconate dehydrogenase reaction by the availability of NADP$^+$. It is thus for example linked to fatty acid synthesis, which consumes NADPH+H$^+$ thereby generating NADP$^+$ and stimulating the pathway.

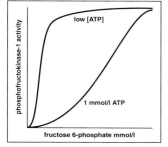

Diagram 12.1. Graph showing that ATP inhibits phosphofructokinase-1, and that this inhibition is overcome by increased concentrations of fructose 6-phosphate.

Diagram 12.2. Pentose phosphate pathway in red blood cells. Red blood cells, which contain oxygen in high concentrations, are vulnerable to oxidative damage caused by peroxides. This is prevented by glutathione peroxidase, which needs **reduced** glutathione (GSH) which is regenerated from **oxidized** gluthathione (GSSG) and NADPH+H$^+$ formed in the pentose phosphate pathway.

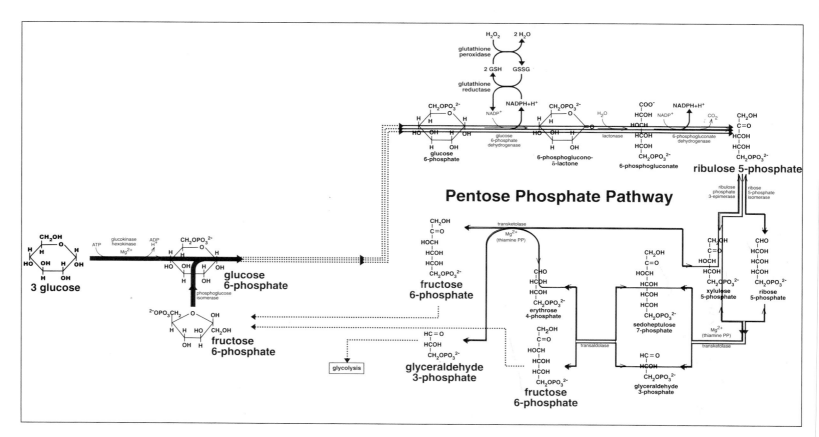

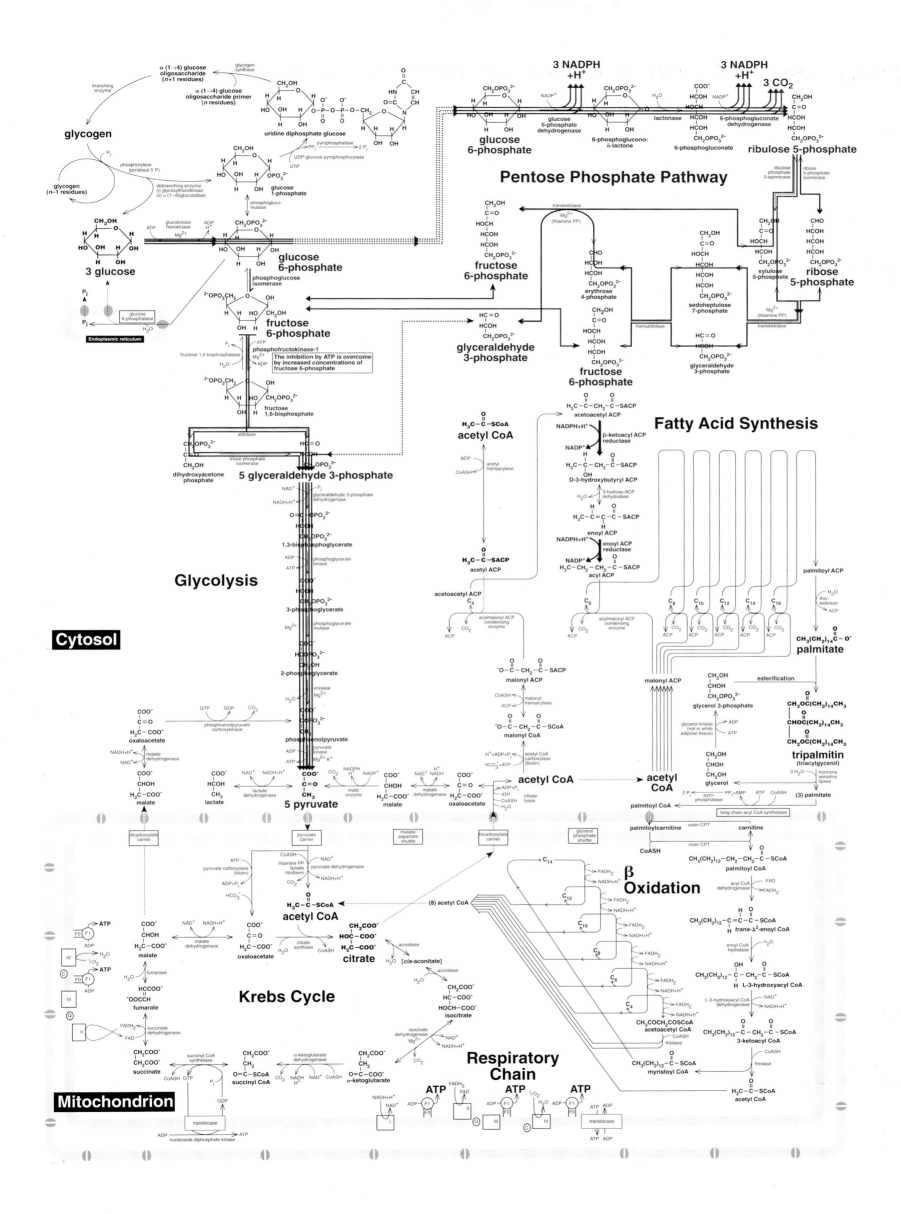

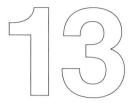

The pyruvate/malate cycle

The pyruvate/malate cycle has two main functions associated with lipogenesis: it transports acetyl CoA units from the mitochondrion into the cytosol, and it generates NADPH+H $^+$ in the reaction catalysed by the **malic enzyme**.

Chart 13: The pyruvate/malate cycle

Fatty acid synthesis occurs in the cytosol. However, the carbon source, i.e. acetyl CoA, is produced by pyruvate dehydrogenase in the mitochondrion. Transport of acetyl CoA from the mitochondrion into the cytosol involves the **pyruvate/malate cycle**.

The principal stages are:

1 One molecule of pyruvate is carboxylated by pyruvate carboxylase to form **oxaloacetate**.

2 A second pyruvate molecule forms **acetyl CoA** by the pyruvate dehydrogenase reaction.

3 The acetyl CoA and oxaloacetate so formed condense to form citrate which is transported to the cytosol for cleavage by citrate lyase to oxaloacetate and **acetyl CoA** for lipogenesis. Oxaloacetate is reduced by cytoso-

Chart 13 opposite. The pyruvate/malate cycle.

Diagram 13.1. Lactate as a substrate for fatty acid synthesis.

lic malate dehydrogenase and **malate** is formed. Malate is oxidatively decarboxylated by the **malic enzyme (malate dehydrogenase, decarboxylating)** with the formation of NADPH+H $^+$, CO $_2$ and pyruvate, thus completing the cycle.

The relative contributions of the pentose phosphate pathway and the pyruvate/malate cycle to the provision of NADPH+H $^+$ for fatty acid synthesis

For each acetyl unit added to the acyl ACP chain during the process of fatty acid synthesis, two molecules of NADPH+H $^+$ are needed (see Chapter 11).

Experimental evidence suggests that if glucose is used for fatty acid synthesis, the pentose phosphate pathway supplies 60% of the NADPH+H $^+$ needed with 40% produced by the pyruvate/malate cycle.

Fatty acid synthesis is also possible from other precursors e.g. amino acids (see Chapter 21) or lactate (see Diagram 13.1). For instance, if lactate is used for fatty acid synthesis, only 25% of the NADPH+H $^+$ needed is provided by the pyruvate/malate cycle.

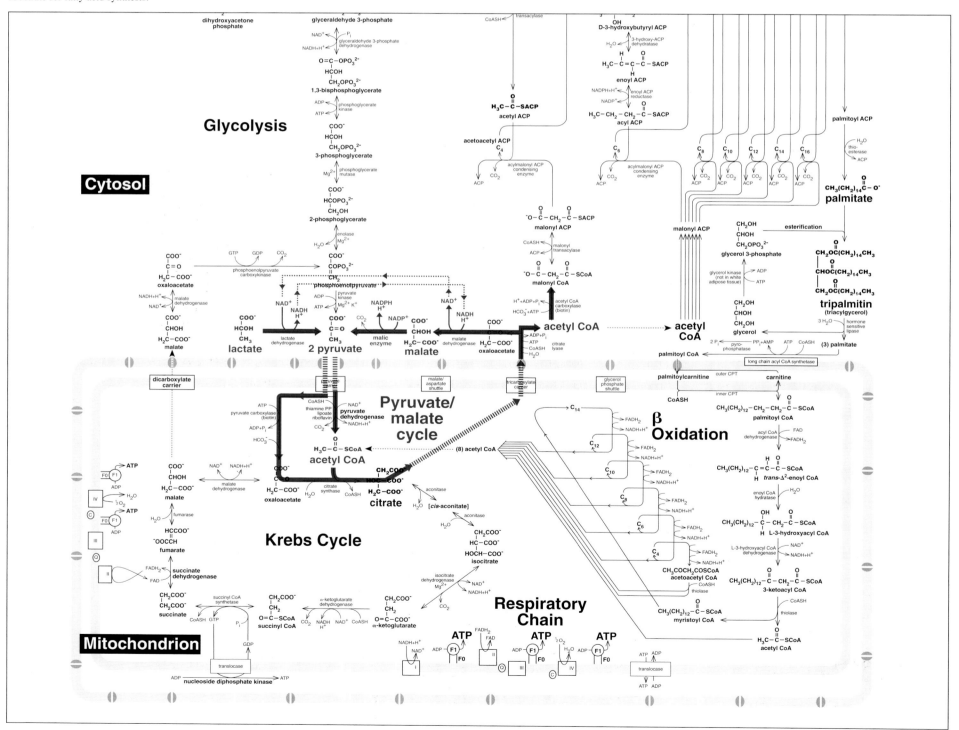

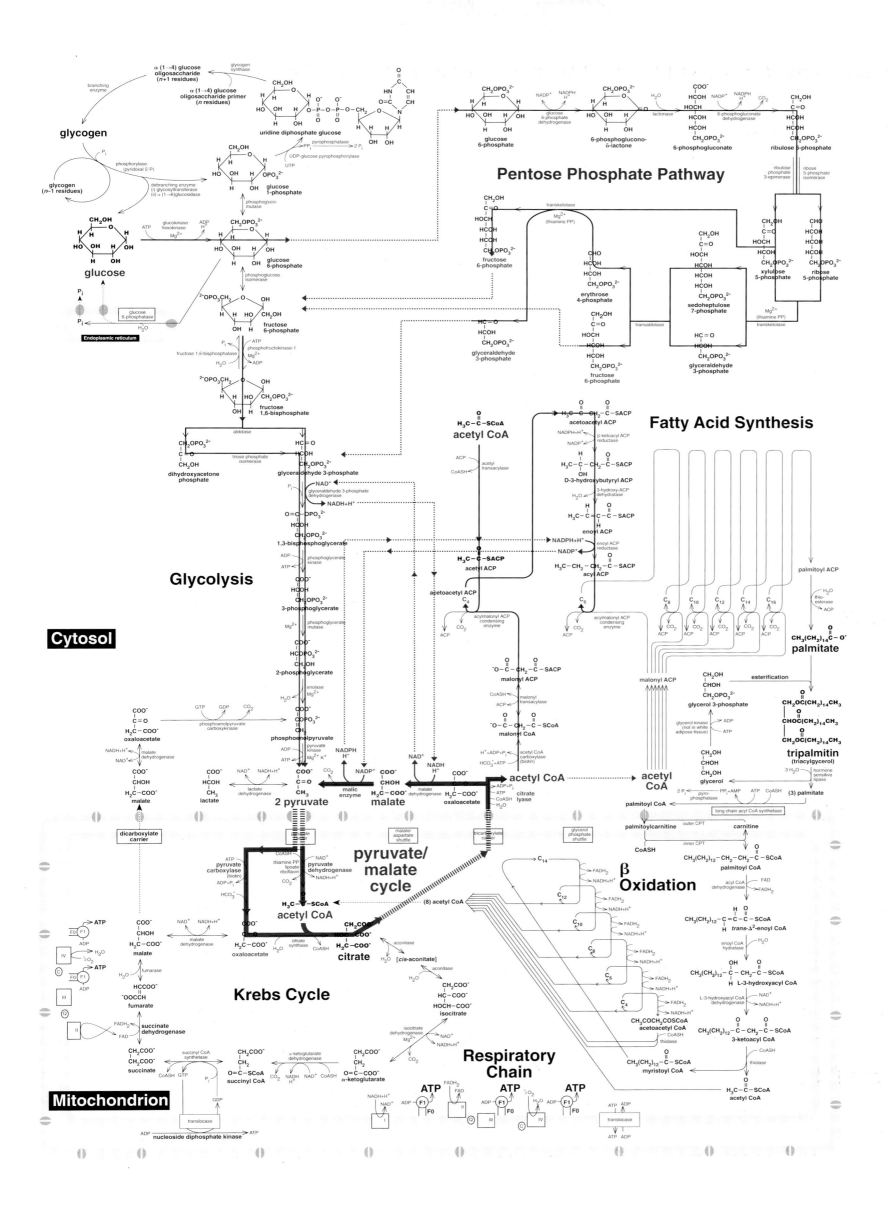

Mammals cannot synthesize glucose from fatty acids

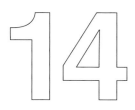

14

Fatty acids cannot be used as a gluconeogenic precursor by mammals for the reasons explained below. Since glucose is a vital fuel for brain and red blood cells, this presents a serious difficulty during prolonged starvation once the glycogen reserves have been depleted (although the brain can adapt to use ketone bodies as a respiratory fuel). It is unfortunate that, because the fatty acids derived from triacylglycerol in adipose tissue cannot be used for gluconeogenesis, muscle proteins must be degraded to maintain glucose homoeostasis in the starving state, thereby causing wasting of the skeletal muscles.

Chart 14.1 below. Two molecules of carbon dioxide are evolved when acetyl CoA is oxidized in the Krebs cycle.

Chart 14.1: Two molecules of carbon dioxide are evolved when acetyl CoA is oxidized in the Krebs cycle

The chart illustrates why mammals cannot convert fatty acids to glucose. Fatty acids are oxidized to acetyl CoA. Because the pyruvate dehydrogenase

and pyruvate kinase reactions are irreversible, acetyl CoA cannot simply be carboxylated to pyruvate and proceed to form glucose by reversal of glycolysis. Instead, the two carbon atoms contained in the acetyl group of acetyl CoA enter the Krebs cycle. However, two carbon atoms are removed as carbon dioxide as shown in the chart. Hence, in animals, there can be no **net** synthesis of glucose from acetyl CoA. Having emphasized this point, it should be noted that if fatty acids which are uniformly labelled with ^{14}C are fed to mammals, some of the radioactive label does become incorporated into glucose. This is because the ^{14}C-fatty acid is catabolized to ^{14}C-acetyl CoA which enters the Krebs cycle. The label is incorporated into citrate and may be retained in the other intermediates of the cycle. If ^{14}C-malate is formed, it can leave the mitchondrion and the ^{14}C label may be incorporated into glucose by gluconeogenesis. **NB:** This incorporation of ^{14}C-label from acetyl CoA into carbohydrate does not represent **net** synthesis because two carbon atoms have been lost as carbon dioxide in the process.

Glycerol derived from triacylglycerol can be used for glucose synthesis

When the triacylglycerol stored in adipose tissue is hydrolysed by hormone-sensitive lipase, fatty acids and glycerol are released. Unlike fatty acids, glycerol **can** be used for glucose synthesis by the liver (see Chapter 31). Glycerol is transported in the blood to the liver, where it is phosphorylated by glycerol kinase to glycerol 3-phosphate, which is reduced to dihydroxy-acetone phosphate, two molecules of which are converted to glucose, as shown in Chart 14.1.

Possible gluconeogenic pathways using fatty acid precursors in mammals

Draye and Vamecq have challenged the standard textbook dogma that mammals are unable to convert fatty acids to glucose. They point out that fatty acids with an odd number of carbon atoms, and branched-chain fatty acids, can be metabolized to produce succinyl CoA. Moreover ω-oxidation of even-numbered fatty acids yields succinate. Both of these products are gluconeogenic precursors. However, gluconeogenesis from these fatty acids is unlikely to be quantitatively significant in physiological terms.

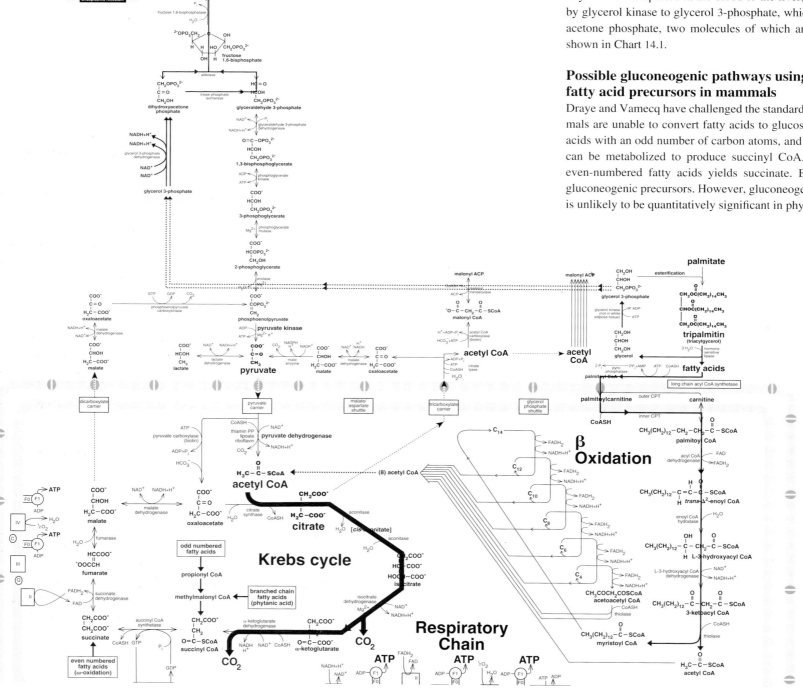

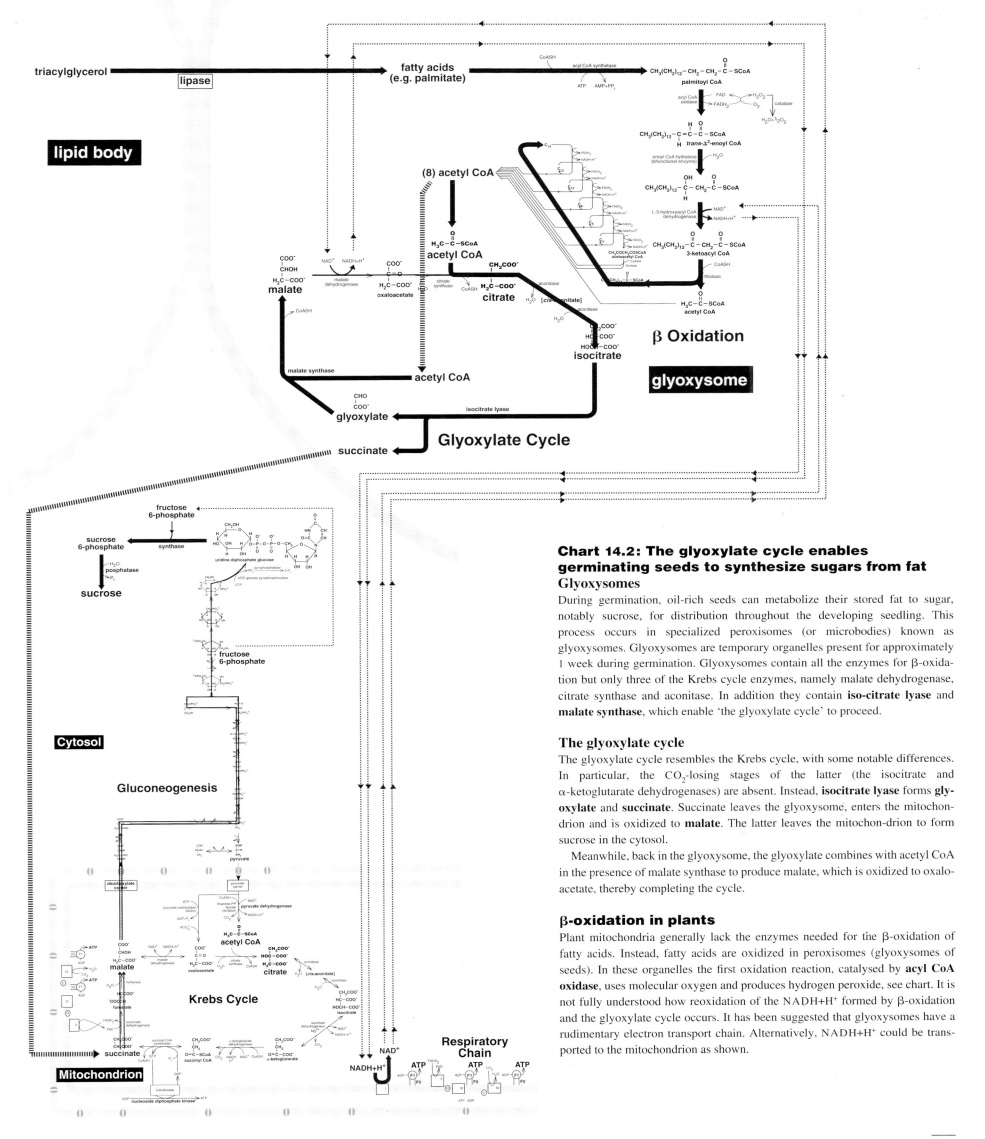

Chart 14.2: The glyoxylate cycle enables germinating seeds to synthesize sugars from fat

Glyoxysomes

During germination, oil-rich seeds can metabolize their stored fat to sugar, notably sucrose, for distribution throughout the developing seedling. This process occurs in specialized peroxisomes (or microbodies) known as glyoxysomes. Glyoxysomes are temporary organelles present for approximately 1 week during germination. Glyoxysomes contain all the enzymes for β-oxidation but only three of the Krebs cycle enzymes, namely malate dehydrogenase, citrate synthase and aconitase. In addition they contain **iso-citrate lyase** and **malate synthase**, which enable 'the glyoxylate cycle' to proceed.

The glyoxylate cycle

The glyoxylate cycle resembles the Krebs cycle, with some notable differences. In particular, the CO_2-losing stages of the latter (the isocitrate and α-ketoglutarate dehydrogenases) are absent. Instead, **isocitrate lyase** forms **glyoxylate** and **succinate**. Succinate leaves the glyoxysome, enters the mitochondrion and is oxidized to **malate**. The latter leaves the mitochondrion to form sucrose in the cytosol.

Meanwhile, back in the glyoxysome, the glyoxylate combines with acetyl CoA in the presence of malate synthase to produce malate, which is oxidized to oxaloacetate, thereby completing the cycle.

β-oxidation in plants

Plant mitochondria generally lack the enzymes needed for the β-oxidation of fatty acids. Instead, fatty acids are oxidized in peroxisomes (glyoxysomes of seeds). In these organelles the first oxidation reaction, catalysed by **acyl CoA oxidase**, uses molecular oxygen and produces hydrogen peroxide, see chart. It is not fully understood how reoxidation of the $NADH+H^+$ formed by β-oxidation and the glyoxylate cycle occurs. It has been suggested that glyoxysomes have a rudimentary electron transport chain. Alternatively, $NADH+H^+$ could be transported to the mitochondrion as shown.

Metabolism of triacylglycerol to provide energy as ATP

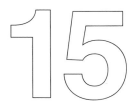

Fatty acids are oxidized and ATP is formed

Fatty acids are an important respiratory fuel for many tissues, especially muscle. The complete oxidation of a typical fatty acid, palmitate, is shown in Chart 15.

Chart 15: The oxidation of fatty acids with energy conserved as ATP

Three metabolic pathways are involved. These are: the **β-oxidation pathway**, **Krebs cycle** and the **respiratory chain**. First of all fatty acids must be liberated from **triacylglycerol** by **hormone-sensitive lipase**. The chart shows the hydrolysis of tripalmitin to yield three molecules of **palmitate** and one molecule of **glycerol**. Next, **palmitoyl CoA** is formed in a reaction catalysed by **long chain acyl CoA synthetase**; ATP is consumed in the process and AMP (adenosine monosphosphate) and inorganic pyrophos-

Chart 15 opposite. Metabolism of triacylglycerol to provide energy as ATP.

phate (PP$_i$) are formed. Thus energy equal to two ATP equivalents is required for this activation reaction. The palmitoyl CoA formed is transported into the mitochondrion using the carnitine shuttle (Chapter 33). Once in the mitochondrial matrix it is successively oxidized and cleaved to yield eight 2-carbon fragments of acetyl CoA by the β-oxidation pathway. For each turn of the β-oxidation cycle, one FADH$_2$ and one NADH+H$^+$ are formed, i.e. seven FADH$_2$ and seven NADH+H$^+$ are formed from palmitate. The eight molecules of acetyl CoA then enter the Krebs cycle, where they are oxidized as shown.

The NADH+H$^+$ and FADH$_2$ formed by both of these pathways are oxidized by the respiratory chain and yield a total of 123 ATP by oxidative phosphorylation. A further eight ATP are derived from the GTP molecules produced by substrate-level phosphorylation in the Krebs cycle.

By inspecting the chart, we can now take stock of the ATP yield from one molecule of palmitate:

From β-oxidation	ATP yield
By oxidative phosphorylation of 7 FADH$_2$	14
By oxidative phosphorylation of 7 NADH+H$^+$	21
	35 ATP

From Krebs cycle	ATP yield
By substrate-level phosphorylation via GTP	8
By oxidative phosphorylation of 8 FADH$_2$	16
By oxidative phosphorylation of 24 NADH+H$^+$	72
	96 ATP

The total yield is therefore 35+96=131 ATP. We must remember, however, to subtract the two ATP equivalents consumed in the initial acyl CoA synthetase reaction. **Therefore the net yield from the oxidation of one molecule of palmitate is 129 molecules of ATP.**

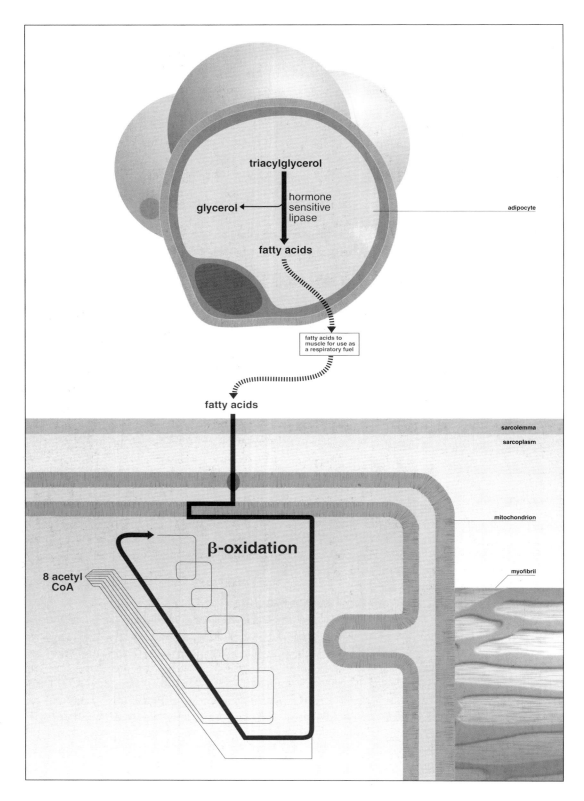

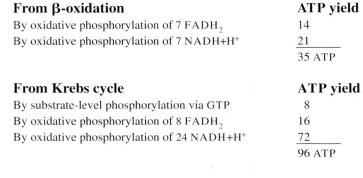

Diagram 15.1. When energy is required under conditions of stress such as 'fight or flight', exercise or starvation, the hormones adrenaline and glucagon stimulate triacylglycerol mobilization by activating hormone-sensitive lipase (Chapter 32), and fatty acids and glycerol are released. The fatty acids are bound to albumin and transported in the blood to the tissues for oxidation, e.g. by muscle. The glycerol is converted by the liver to glucose (Chapter 31), which in turn is released for oxidation, especially by the red blood cells and brain, neither of which can use fatty acids as a respiratory fuel.

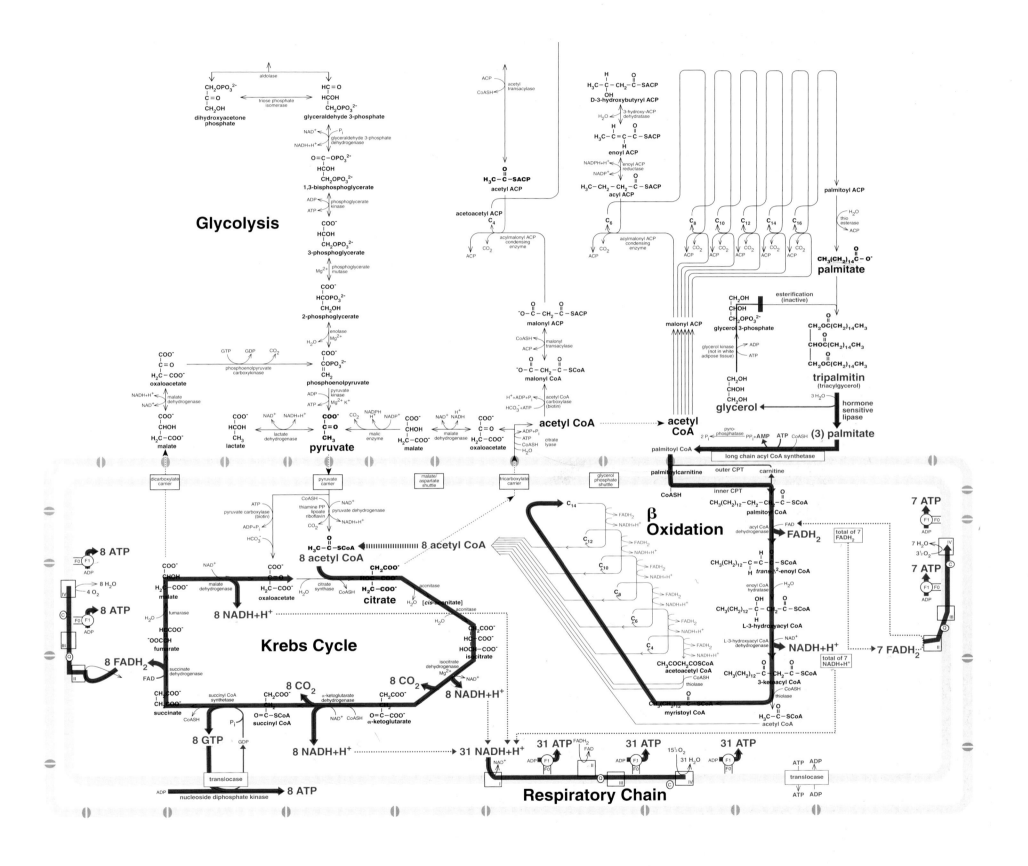

The ornithine cycle for the production of urea: 'the urea cycle'

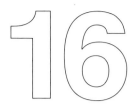

A study of the other metabolic cycle elucidated by Krebs, the 'Krebs–Henseleit ornithine cycle' popularly (but inaccurately) known as the 'urea cycle', offers an overview of amino acid metabolism. In the well-fed state, any amino acids surplus to requirement for protein synthesis can be metabolized to non-nitrogenous substances such as glucose, glycogen or fatty acids; or they can be oxidized to generate ATP. On the other hand, during fasting or starvation, catabolic wasting of muscle occurs thereby yielding amino acids which are used for gluconeogenesis so as to maintain normoglycaemia. Because the ammonia derived from these amino acids is extremely toxic, it is converted to non-toxic **urea** for urinary excretion. Any ammonia which evades detoxification as urea can alternatively be incorporated into glutamine by glutamine synthetase, which has been described by Häussinger as serving as a scavenger for stray ammonium ions.

The origins of the nitrogen used for urea synthesis

In the well-fed state, amino acids are formed from dietary proteins by proteolytic digestion in the gastrointestinal tract. The amino acids are then absorbed into the bloodstream and may be used intact for protein synthesis. Alternatively, surplus amino acids can be metabolized to glucose, be used for fatty acid synthesis, or be catabolized to generate ATP. The amino groups are removed by transamination and deamination prior to urea synthesis in the periportal hepatocytes. The residual carbon skeletons are metabolized to the gluconeogenic precursors: pyruvate, succinyl CoA, fumarate, α-ketoglutarate, oxaloacetate; or alternatively to the ketone bodies or their precursors (see Chapters 20 and 34).

In starvation, the circulating amino acids are derived mainly from proteolysis of muscle protein. Transamination of the amino acids (particularly the branched-chain amino acids isoleucine, valine and leucine) occurs in the muscle in partnership with pyruvate, so that the amino acid pool in the venous blood draining from the muscle is enriched with alanine (see Chapter 18). This alanine is transported to the liver, entering via the hepatic artery system, where transamination with α-ketoglutarate occurs to form glutamate.

Chart 16: Nitrogen, in the form of ammonium ions or glutamate, is used for urea synthesis

As shown in Chart 16, amino acids, whether of dietary or endogenous (muscle) origin, enter the pathway for urea synthesis by the **transdeamination route** or the **transamination route**.

Transdeamination route

This route consists of an initial transamination in the cytosol, followed by deamination in the mitochondrion. Initially **α-ketoglutarate** accepts an amino group from the donor amino acid to form **glutamate** in a cytosolic reaction catalysed by an **aminotransferase.** The glutamate is then transported into the mitochondrion by the glutamate carrier where it is oxidatively deaminated by **glutamate dehydrogenase** to form α-ketoglutarate and **ammonium ions**. The ammonium is incorporated into **carbamoyl phosphate**, which in turn reacts with **ornithine** to enter the urea cycle as **citrulline**.

Transamination route

Alternatively, amino acid nitrogen can enter the urea cycle via the transamination route, which involves two transamination reactions. Again, α-ketoglutarate initially accepts the amino group from the donor amino acid and once again glutamate is formed as described above. However, a second transamination now follows, with oxaloacetate accepting the amino group from glutamate to form **aspartate** in a reaction catalysed by **aspartate aminotransferase (AST)**. This aspartate now carries the second amino group into the urea cycle by condensing with **citrulline** to form **arginosuccinate**. Arginosuccinate is then cleaved to form **fumarate** and **arginine**. Finally, arginine is hydrolysed to **ornithine** and **urea**, and ornithine is regenerated for another rotation of the cycle.

What happens to the fumarate produced by the arginosuccinate lyase reaction? Confusion in the textbooks!

This text is designed as a companion to existing textbooks of biochemistry, and so a dilemma occurs if some of these hitherto faithful companions disagree among themselves while others maintain a discreet silence. Such a dilemma arises with the fate of the fumarate produced from arginosuccinate. There is general agreement that it is metabolized to malate, but the details of the subcellular location of this transformation vary. The reactions are:

$$\text{fumarate} \underset{\text{fumarase}}{\overset{H_2O}{\rightleftharpoons}} \text{malate} \underset{\substack{\text{malate} \\ \text{dehydrogenase}}}{\overset{NAD^+ \quad \overset{NADH}{H^+}}{\rightleftharpoons}} \text{oxaloacetate} \underset{\substack{\text{aspartate} \\ \text{aminotransferase}}}{\overset{\text{glutamate} \quad \overset{\alpha\text{-ketoglutarate}}{}}{\rightleftharpoons}} \text{aspartate}$$

Whereas some of the textbooks avoid reference to the subcellular distribution of these enzymes, others indicate that the reactions take place in the mitochondrion, and others suggest they occur in the cytosol. The latter concept has been incorporated in this edition and is supported by Tuboi *et al.*, who have shown that fumarase is found in both the cytosol and mitochondrion in rat liver. It is possible, therefore, that the fumarate cleaved from arginosuccinate is hydrated to form malate in the cytosol. The malate is subsequently oxidized to oxaloacetate by cytosolic malate dehydrogenase. Finally, oxaloacetate accepts an amino group from glutamate to form aspartate, thus completing an entirely cytosolic transamination route for entry of the nitrogen into the urea cycle.

The purine nucleotide cycle

The purine nucleotide cycle described by Lowenstein, although present in many types of tissues, is particularly active in muscle. During vigorous exercise in rats, the blood concentration of ammonium ions can increase five-fold. This ammonium is thought to be derived from aspartate via the purine nucleotide cycle. This cycle is mentioned again in Chapter 30.

References

Häussinger D., Glutamine metabolism in the liver: overview and current concepts. *Metabolism* **38**, 14–17, 1989.

Tuboi S., Suzuki T., Sato M. and Yoshida T., Rat liver mitochondrial and cytosolic fumarases with identical amino acid sequences are encoded from a single mRNA with two alternative in-phase AUG-initiation sites. *Adv Enzyme Regul* **30**, 289–303, 1990.

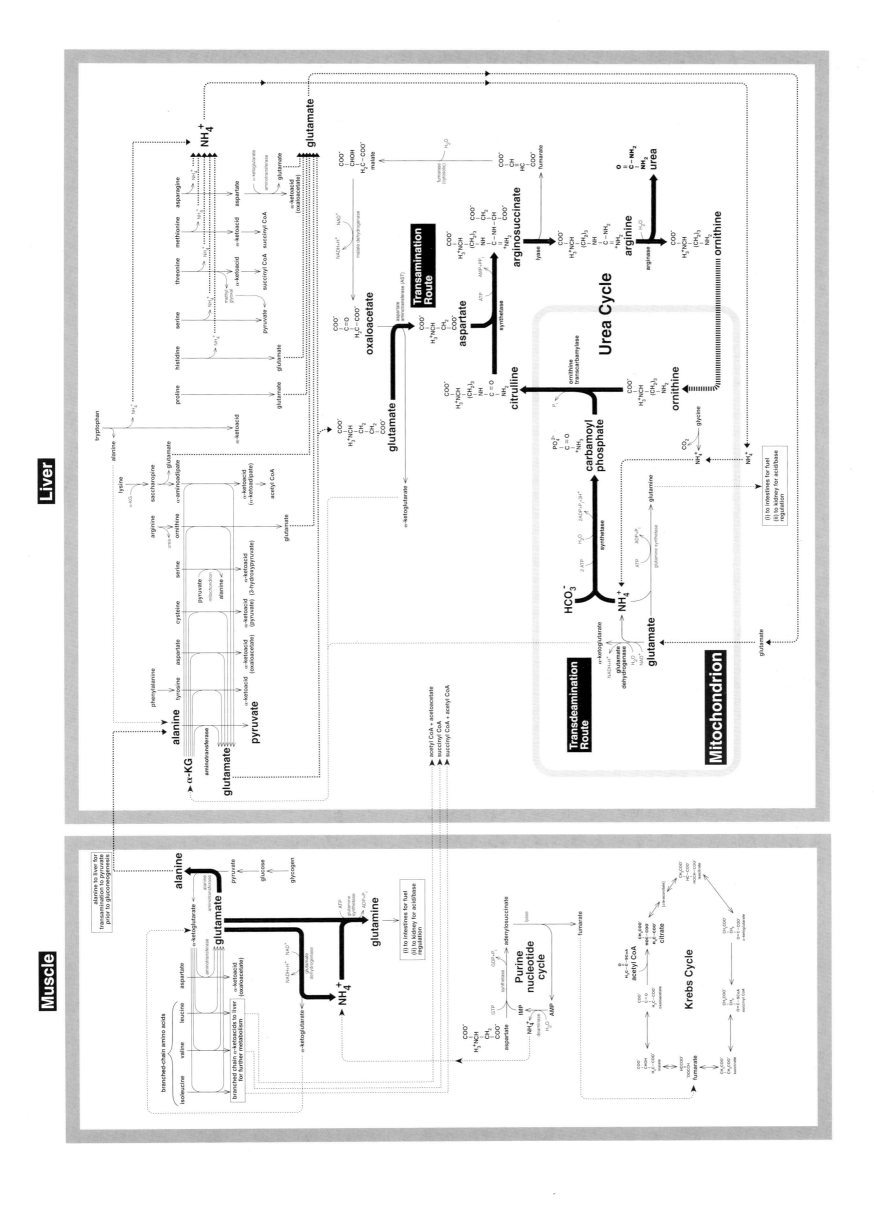

Biosynthesis of the non-essential amino acids

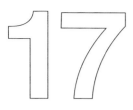

Chart 17 opposite. Biosynthesis of the non-essential amino acids.

Whereas plants and some bacteria are capable of synthesizing all of the amino acids necessary for the formation of cellular proteins and other vital molecules, this is not the case in mammals. Mammals, including humans, can synthesize only 11 of these amino acids, namely tyrosine, aspartate, asparagine, alanine, serine, glycine, cysteine, glutamate, glutamine, proline and arginine. These are known as the **non-essential amino acids** and their biosynthesis is shown in chart 17. On the other hand, the other nine amino acids: phenylalanine, threonine, methionine, lysine, tryptophan, leucine, isoleucine, valine and histidine cannot be synthesized. They are known as the **essential amino acids**.

Tyrosine
Biosynthesis. Tyrosine is formed from the essential amino acid phenylalanine in the presence of phenylalanine monooxygenase.

Uses. Tyrosine is a precursor in the synthesis of adrenaline, noradrenaline, thyroxine and the pigment, melanin.

Serine, glycine and cysteine
These amino acids are made from intermediates formed by glycolysis.

Biosynthesis of serine. Serine is synthesized by a pathway commonly known as 'the phosphorylated pathway'. First, 3-phosphoglycerate is oxidized to 3-phosphohydroxypyruvate, which is then transaminated to 3-phosphoserine. Finally, hydrolysis by a specific phosphatase yields serine. This phosphoserine phosphatase is inhibited by serine providing feedback regulation of the pathway. (**NB:** The so-called 'non-phosphorylated pathway' for serine metabolism is important in the gluconeogenic state, see Chapter 20).

Uses. Serine is a component of the phospholipid, phosphatidylserine.

Biosynthesis of glycine. Glycine can be formed by two routes, both of which involve serine. Glycine is formed from serine by a reversible reaction catalysed by **serine hydroxymethyltransferase**. This enzyme uses the coenzyme tetrahydrofolate (THF), which is formed by reduction of the vitamin folic acid (see Chapter 23). It accepts a 1-carbon fragment from serine to form N^5,N^{10}-methylene tetrahydrofolate, and glycine is formed.

An alternative route for glycine synthesis uses CO_2 and NH_4^+ in a reaction catalysed by the mitochondrial enzyme **glycine synthase** (also known as the glycine cleavage enzyme when working in the reverse direction, see Chapter 19). The second carbon atom is derived from N^5,N^{10}-methylene THF obtained from serine in the previously mentioned reaction catalysed by serine hydroxymethyltransferase.

Uses. The demand for glycine by the body is considerable, and it has been estimated that the requirement for endogenous synthesis of glycine is between 10 and 50 times the dietary intake. Apart from its contribution to cellular proteins, glycine is required for the synthesis of purines, collagen, porphyrins, bile salts, creatine and glutathione. Glycine can also be conjugated with certain drugs and toxic substances to facilitate their excretion in the urine. Finally, glycine is made by mitochondria in the brain, where it acts as an inhibitory neurotransmitter. Hypotheses have implicated a deficiency of serine hydroxymethyltransferase with schizophrenia.

Biosynthesis of cysteine. Cysteine can be formed from serine provided that the essential amino acid methionine is available to donate a sulphur atom.

When there is a metabolic demand for cysteine, homocysteine condenses with serine to yield cystathionine in a reaction catalysed by cystathionine synthase. Cystathionine is then cleaved by cystathionase to release cysteine.

Uses. Cysteine is a component of the tripeptide, glutathione (γ-glutamylcysteinylglycine).

Aspartate and asparagine
Biosynthesis of aspartate. Aspartate is readily formed by the transamination of oxaloacetate by glutamate in the presence of aspartate aminotransferase (AST).

Uses. Aspartate is an amino donor in urea synthesis, and in both pyrimidine and purine synthesis.

Biosynthesis of asparagine. Asparagine is synthesized by amide transfer from glutamine in the presence of aspartate synthetase.

Uses. Asparagine is incorporated into cellular proteins but appears to have no other role in mammals. However, although animal cells can usually synthesize sufficient asparagine for their requirements, this is not so for some rapidly dividing leukaemic cells, which obtain their asparagine from the blood. Treatment of leukaemic patients with the enzyme asparaginase depletes the plasma of asparagine, thereby depriving the neoplastic cells of this vital amino acid and restricting their growth.

Glutamate, glutamine, proline and arginine
These amino acids are formed from the Krebs cycle intermediate, α-ketoglutarate.

Biosynthesis of glutamate. Glutamate is formed by the reductive amination of α-ketoglutarate by glutamate dehydrogenase.

Biosynthesis of glutamine. Glutamine is formed from glutamate and NH_4^+ in an ATP-requiring reaction catalysed by glutamine synthetase.

Uses. Glutamine is a very important source of nitrogen for purine and pyrimidine (and hence nucleic acid) synthesis (see Chapters 23 and 24). Glutamine also is important in regulating pH in acidotic conditions.

Biosynthesis of proline. In the presence of pyrroline 5-carboxylate synthetase, glutamate is converted to glutamate γ-semialdehyde, which spontaneously cyclizes to pyrroline 5-carboxylate. This can then be reduced to proline.

Biosynthesis of arginine. Pyrroline 5-carboxylate is in equilibrium with glutamate γ-semialdehyde, which can be transaminated by ornithine transaminase to yield ornithine. Ornithine can then enter the urea cycle and so form arginine (see Chapter 16).

Uses. Arginine is an intermediate in the urea cycle. It is also the source of the vasodilator, nitric oxide.

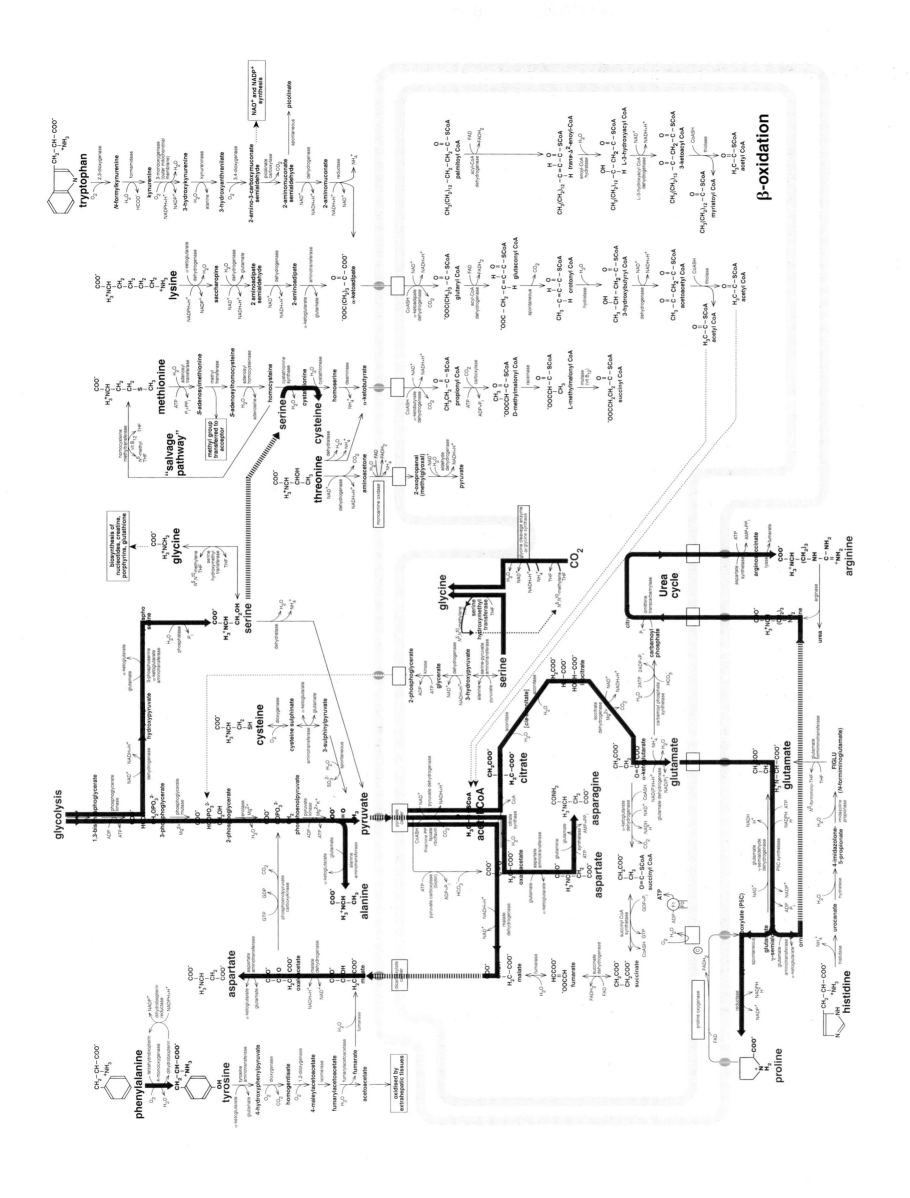

Catabolism of amino acids, part I

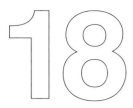

Chart 18 opposite. Formation of alanine and glutamine by muscle.

Proteins, whether of dietary origin in the well-fed state or derived from muscle protein in starvation, can be degraded to amino acids for direct oxidation as a respiratory fuel with the generation of ATP. However, it is also possible that in the well-fed state amino acids may first of all be converted to glycogen or triacylglycerol for fuel storage prior to energy metabolism. Alternatively, in starvation, certain glucogenic amino acids are initially converted to alanine in muscle, which is subsequently converted by the liver to glucose to provide fuel for the brain and red blood cells. Finally, the ketogenic amino acids form the ketone bodies, which are a valuable fuel for the brain in starvation.

The catabolism of aspartate and the branched-chain amino acids (BCAAs) will be emphasized here, and catabolism of the remaining amino acids will be described in Chapter 19.

Dietary protein as a source of energy in the well-fed state

Protein is digested in the gastrointestinal tract to release its 20 constituent amino acids. If they are surplus to the body's requirement for incorporation into proteins or other essential molecules derived from amino acids, they may be metabolized to glycogen or fat (see Chapters 20 and 21) and subsequently used for energy metabolism. Alternatively, they can be oxidized directly as a metabolic fuel. However, different tissues have different abilities to catabolize the various amino acids.

Metabolism of muscle protein during starvation or prolonged exercise

In the well-fed state, muscle uses glucose and fatty acids for energy metabolism. However, during fasting, starvation or prolonged exercise, protein from muscle plays an important role in glucose homoeostasis. For example, during an overnight fast the hepatic glycogen reserves can be depleted and life-threatening hypoglycaemia must be prevented. Remember that fat cannot be converted to glucose (see Chapter 14), apart from the glycerol derived from triacylglycerol metabolism. Consequently, muscle tissue remains as the only glucogenic source and must be 'sacrificed' to maintain blood glucose concentrations and thus ensure a vital supply of energy for the red blood cells and the brain.

During starvation, muscle protein must first be broken down into its constituent amino acids, but the details of intracellular proteolysis are still not fully understood. It was once thought that, following proteolysis, all of the different amino acids were released from the muscle into the blood in proportion to their composition in muscle proteins. Research has shown that this idea is more complicated than originally supposed. During fasting, the blood draining from muscle is especially enriched with alanine and glutamine which can each constitute up to 30% of the total amino acids released by muscle, a proportion greatly in excess of their relative abundance in muscle proteins. Alanine released from muscle is taken up by the liver in a process known as the **alanine cycle**. Glutamine is not taken up by the liver, but is used by the intestines as a fuel, and by the kidney for gluconeogenesis and pH homoeostasis.

Catabolism of the branched-chain amino acids (BCAAs)

The oxidation of the branched-chain amino acids (leucine, isoleucine and valine) is shown in Chart 18. The branched-chain α-ketoacid dehydrogenase (BCKADH) resembles pyruvate dehydrogenase. Moreover, the oxidation of the acyl CoA derivatives formed by this reaction has many similarities with the β-oxidation of fatty acids, which is included in Chart 18 for the purpose of comparison. **NB:** Not all tissues can oxidize the BCAAs. Whereas muscle has BCAA aminotransferase activity, liver lacks this enzyme. However, liver has BCKADH activity and can oxidize the branched-chain ketoacids.

It should be noted that, in starvation and diabetes, the activity of muscle BCKADH is increased up to fivefold, thereby promoting oxidation of the BCAAs in muscle.

Chart 18: Formation of alanine and glutamine by muscle
Alanine and the alanine cycle
The alanine cycle was proposed by Felig, who demonstrated increased production of alanine by muscle during starvation. The BCAAs are the major donors of amino groups for alanine synthesis. Pyruvate, for transamination to alanine, can be formed from isoleucine and valine (via succinyl CoA), from certain other amino acids, e.g. aspartate, or alternatively, from glycolysis. The alanine so formed is exported from muscle and is transported via the hepatic artery to the liver, where it is used for gluconeogenesis (see Diagram 18.1).

Glutamine

Glutamine is the most abundant amino acid in the blood. As shown in Chart 18 (and Chart 16), BCAAs are major donors of the amino groups used to form glutamate, which is further aminated by glutamine synthetase to form glutamine.

The ketogenic amino acids leucine and isoleucine as an energy source

As shown in Chart 18, the entire carbon skeleton of leucine, and carbon fragments from isoleucine, are converted to acetoacetate or to acetyl CoA which can be converted into acetoacetate in the liver (see Chapter 34). The ketone bodies can then be oxidized as a respiratory fuel by extrahepatic tissues, as described in Chapter 35.

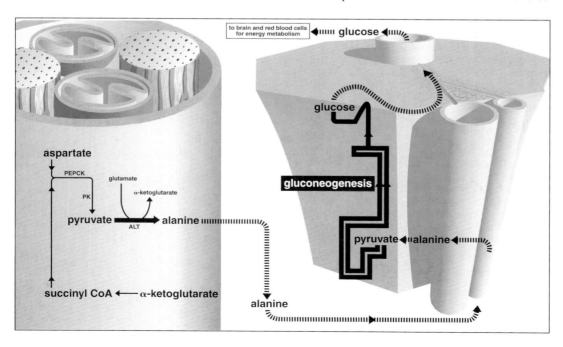

Diagram 18.1.

  Formation of alanine from muscle protein. In starvation, the amino acids derived from muscle protein are degraded to ketoacids. Some of the carbon skeletons from these ketoacids enter Krebs cycle and are metabolized via phosphoenolpyruvate carboxykinase (PEPCK) and pyruvate kinase (PK) to pyruvate. Alanine aminotransferase (ALT) is very active in muscle and so much of the pyruvate produced is transaminated to alanine which leaves the muscle and is transported in the blood to the liver.

  Gluconeogenesis from alanine in the liver. In the liver, alanine is reconverted to pyruvate which is used for gluconeogenesis. **NB:** Pyruvate kinase in the liver is inhibited in the gluconeogenic state both by cyclic AMP-dependent protein phosphorylation, and directly by alanine (see Chapter 31). This prevents the futile recycling of pyruvate which would otherwise happen. The glucose formed can be used for energy metabolism, especially by the brain and red blood cells.

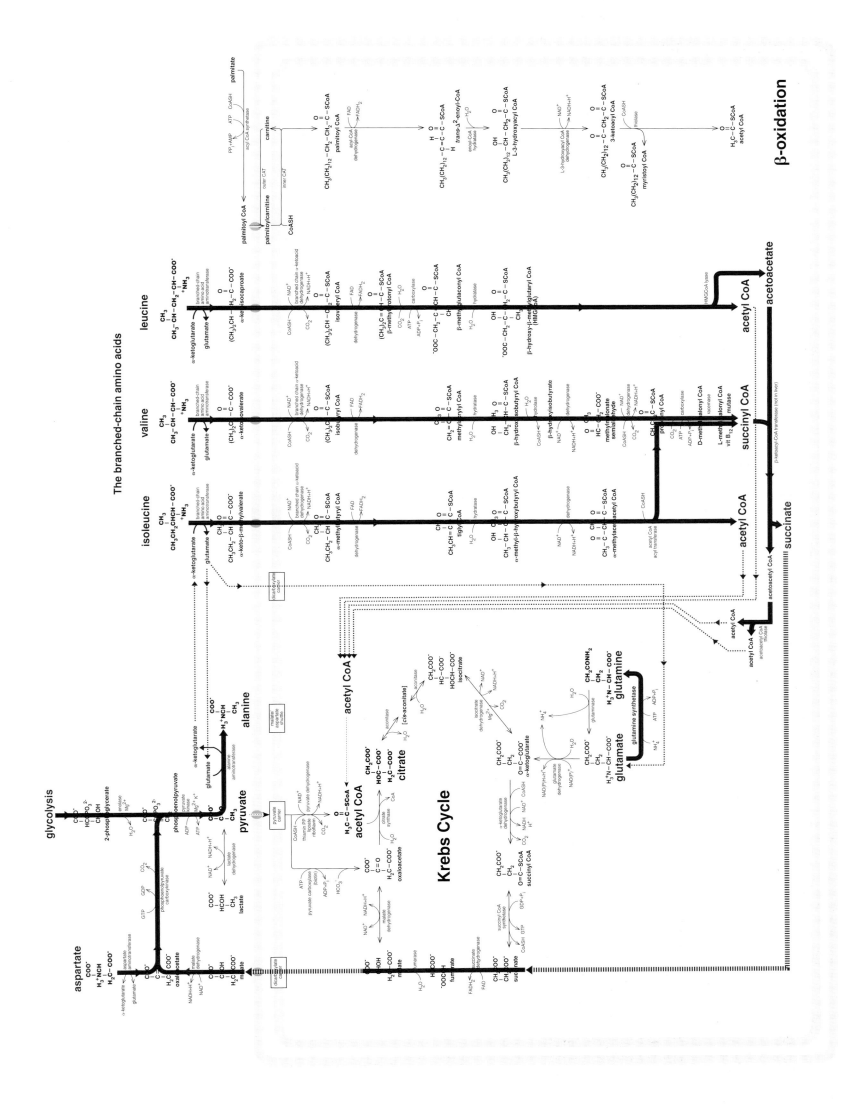

β-oxidation

The branched-chain amino acids

Krebs Cycle

glycolysis

Catabolism of amino acids, part II

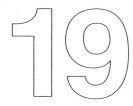

Chart 19 opposite. Catabolism of amino acids, part II.

Diagram 19.1. If amino acids are to be used as a respiratory fuel it is obligatory that their carbon skeletons are converted to acetyl CoA, which must then enter the Krebs cycle for oxidation, producing 12 molecules of ATP as described in Chapter 16. **NB:** The simple entry of the carbon skeletons into Krebs cycle as 'dicarboxylic acids' (α-keto-glutarate, succinate, fumarate or oxaloacetate) does not ensure their complete oxidation for energy metabolism.

Alanine. Alanine is in equilibrium with pyruvate which is oxidatively decarboxylated to CO_2 and acetyl CoA. The latter can then be oxidised in the Krebs cycle.

Glycine. Although there are several possible routes for glycine catabolism, the mitochondrial 'glycine cleavage system' is probably the most important in mammals. This enzyme complex is loosely bound to the mitochondrial inner membrane and has several similarities to the pyruvate dehydrogenase complex. It oxidatively decarboxylates glycine to carbon dioxide and N^5,N^{10}-methylene-tetrahydrofolate (N^5,N^{10}-THF).

Serine. When needed as a respiratory fuel, serine undergoes deamination by serine dehydratase to form pyruvate, as shown in the chart.

Threonine. The most important route for the catabolism of threonine in mammals is the 'aminoacetone pathway'. Threonine dehydrogenase forms the unstable intermediate α-amino-β-ketobutyrate, which is spontaneously decarboxylated to aminoacetone for further catabolism to pyruvate.

It is possible that threonine is also deaminated by serine dehydratase and by a specific threonine dehydratase to form α-ketobutyrate. This could then be metabolized to succinyl CoA, as outlined for methionine metabolism.

Cysteine. There are several possible pathways for cysteine degradation but the most important in mammals is oxidation by cysteine dioxygenase to cysteine sulphinate. This is then transaminated to form 3-sulphinylpyruvate (also known as β-mercaptopyruvate or thiopyruvate), which is converted to pyruvate in a spontaneous reaction.

Methionine. Methionine is activated in an ATP-dependent reaction to form S-adenosylmethionine (SAM), which is the major carrier of methyl groups, beating THF into second place as a donor in biosynthetic methylations. For example, SAM is used in the methylation of noradrenaline to adrenaline by noradrenaline N-methyltransferase. Consequently, the original methionine molecule is demethylated to form S-adenosyl homocysteine, then the adenosyl group is removed to homocysteine. This intermediate can be metabolized in two ways:

1 It can be recycled to methionine in a salvage pathway where the methyl donor is N^5-methyl-THF, using a vitamin B_{12}-dependent reaction catalysed by homocysteine methyltransferase. This is an important pathway which helps to conserve this essential amino acid.

2 It can be degraded to succinyl CoA, which can be further metabolized to pyruvate for energy metabolism.

Lysine. Lysine is unusual in that it cannot be formed from its corresponding α-ketoacid, α-keto-ϵ-aminocaproic acid, which cyclizes to form Δ^1-piperidine-2-carboxylic acid. Degradation of lysine occurs via saccharopine, a compound in which lysine and α-ketoglutarate are bonded as a secondary amine formed with the carbonyl group of α-ketoglutarate and the ϵ-amino group of lysine. Following two further dehydrogenase reactions, α-ketoadipate is formed by transamination. This enters the mitochondrion and is oxidized by a pathway with many similarities to the β-oxidation pathway. Acetoacetyl CoA is formed, thus lysine is classified as a ketogenic amino acid (see Chapter 34).

Tryptophan. Although tryptophan can be oxidized as a respiratory fuel, it is also an important precursor for the synthesis of NAD^+ and $NADP^+$. The regulatory mechanisms involved in the first step of tryptophan catabolism catalysed by tryptophan dioxygenase (also known as tryptophan pyrrolase) have been studied extensively. It is known that the dioxygenase is induced by glucocorticoids, which increase transcription of DNA. Furthermore, glucagon (via cyclic adenosine monophosphate, cAMP) increases the synthesis of dioxygenase by enhancing the translation of mRNA. Hence in starvation, the combined effects of these hormones will promote the oxidation of tryptophan released from muscle protein.

During the catabolism of tryptophan, the amino group is retained in the first three intermediates formed. The amino group in the form of alanine is then hydrolytically cleaved from 3-hydroxykynurenine by kynureninase. This alanine molecule can then be transaminated to pyruvate, thus qualifying tryptophan as a glucogenic amino acid. The other product of kynureninase is 3-hydroxyanthranilate, which is degraded to α-ketoadipate. This is oxidized by a pathway which is similar to β-oxidation to form acetoacetyl CoA. Hence tryptophan is both a ketogenic and a glucogenic amino acid.

Glutamate. This readily enters Krebs cycle following oxidative deamination by glutamate dehydrogenase as α-ketoglutarate. However, for complete oxidation its metabolites must temporarily leave the cycle for conversion to pyruvate. This can then be oxidized to acetyl CoA, which enters the Krebs cycle for energy metabolism, generating 12 molecules of ATP.

Histidine. Histidine is metabolized to glutamate by a pathway which involves the elimination of a 1-carbon group. In this reaction, the formimino group ($-CH=NH$) is transferred from N-formiminoglutamate (FIGLU) to THF, yielding N^5-formimino-THF and glutamate.

Arginine. This amino acid is a constituent of proteins as well as being an intermediate in the urea cycle. Arginine is cleaved by arginase to liberate urea, and ornithine is formed. Ornithine is transaminated by ornithine aminotransferase to form glutamate γ-semialdehyde. The semialdehyde is then oxidized by glutamate γ-semialdehyde dehydrogenase to form glutamate.

Proline. The catabolism of proline to glutamate differs from its biosynthetic pathway. Proline is oxidized by the mitochondrial enzyme proline oxygenase, to form pyrroline 5-carboxylate. This is probably an FAD-dependent enzyme, located in the inner mitochondrial membrane, which can donate electrons directly to cytochrome C in the electron transport chain.

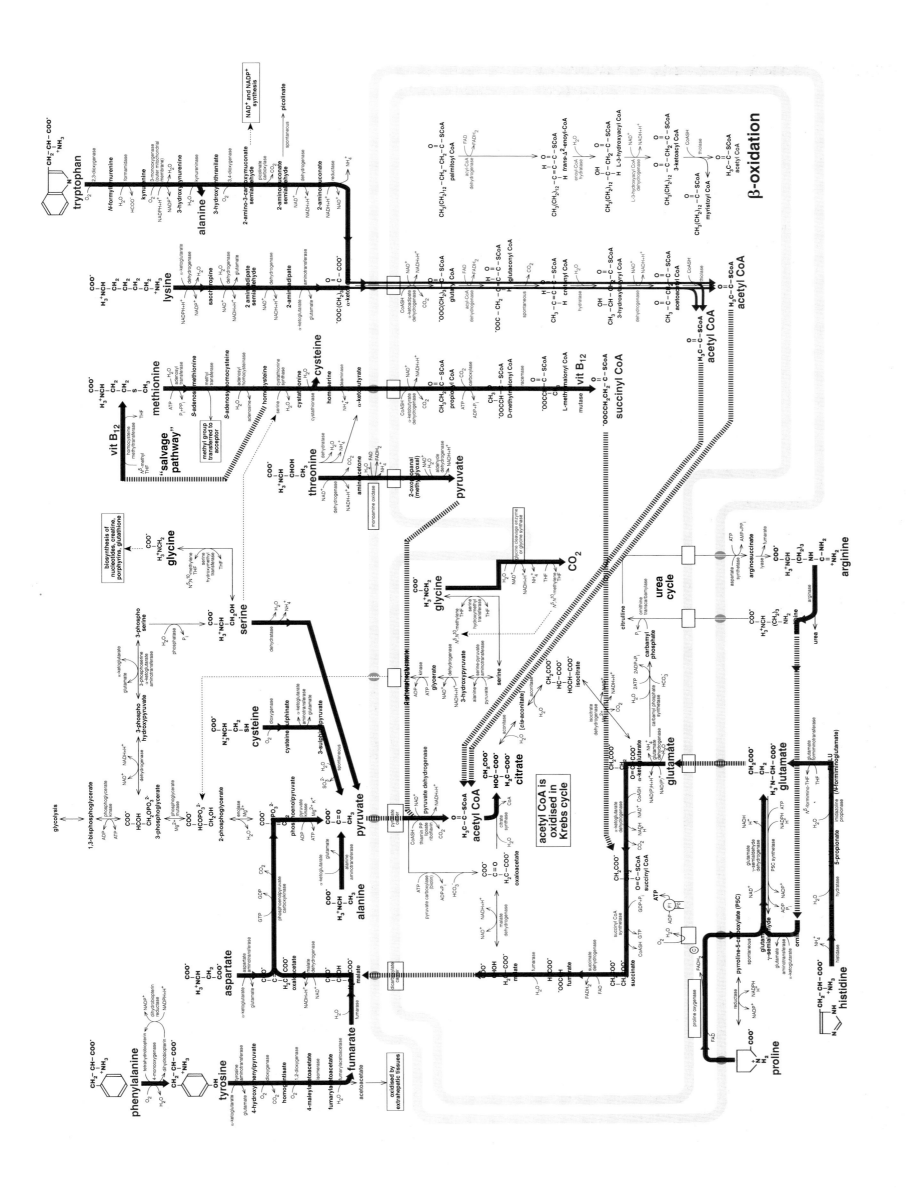

Metabolism of amino acids to glucose in starvation and during the period immediately after refeeding

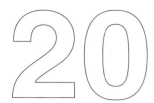

Chart 20 opposite. Gluconeo-genesis from amino acids.

Diagram 20.1. Intermediary metabolism in the early well-fed state. β-Oxidation of fatty acids continues in the early well-fed state. The liver continues in ketogenic and gluconeogenic modes, using lactate (from muscle) and dietary amino acids as gluconeogenic substrates. Muscle uses fatty acids and ketone bodies as respiratory fuels. Also, glycolysis is active in muscle but, since pyruvate dehydrogenase is inactive, lactate is formed.

In liver, the switch from gluconeogenic mode to glycolytic mode in the early well-fed state is a slow process

During starvation, when the glycogen reserves have been exhausted, muscle proteins are degraded to amino acids and used by the liver for gluconeogenesis to maintain the supply of glucose, which is vital for the brain. The important role of alanine as a gluconeogenic precursor is described in Chapter 18.

Following refeeding after a period of starvation, the liver does not switch instantaneously from gluconeogenic to glycolytic mode even though it receives a large glucose load from the intestines. In the early well-fed state the effects of the gluconeogenic and lipolytic hormones linger, and β-oxidation of fatty acids continues. Consequently, large quantities of acetyl CoA are produced which inhibit pyruvate dehydrogenase, thereby favouring gluconeogenesis in the liver. Under these conditions, the amino acids derived from the gastrointestinal digestion of dietary protein can be used for gluconeogenesis, as shown in Chart 20 and described below.

Starvation

In starvation, hepatic gluconeogenesis is active under the hormonal influence of glucagon, cortisol and adrenocorticotropic hormone (ACTH) (see Chapter 31). Glycolysis in the liver is inhibited because glucagon, through cyclic AMP-dependent protein kinase, causes the phosphorylation of hepatic pyruvate kinase, thereby causing inhibition. Moreover, the phosphorylation of hepatic pyruvate kinase is potentiated by its allosteric effector **alanine** (which is abundant in starvation), which therefore further enhances the inhibition of pyruvate kinase.

The role of acetyl CoA in promoting gluconeogenesis in starvation

During starvation, β-oxidation from fatty acids is very active in the liver, and large quantities of acetyl CoA are formed. The accumulated acetyl CoA inhibits pyruvate dehydrogenase and stimulates pyruvate carboxylase. This means that pyruvate (derived from alanine) does not enter Krebs cycle as acetyl CoA, but is instead carboxylated by pyruvate carboxylase to oxaloacetate for metabolism to phosphoenolpyruvate and thence to glucose via gluconeogenesis.

The early well-fed state
Fate of the glucogenic amino acids

During refeeding after a period of starvation, the liver remains in the gluconeogenic mode for a few hours. Consequently, the glucogenic amino acids derived from dietary protein are metabolized to **2-phosphoglycerate** which is their common precursor for gluconeogenesis (see Chart 20 and Diagram 20.1). (**NB:** Evidence suggests that gluconeogenesis from serine originates in the mitochondrion. However, the mitochondrial carriers needed for the route shown, in particular the 2-phosphoglycerate carrier, have not been characterized.) In any event, 2-phosphoglycerate is metabolized to glucose 6-phosphate, which can be used to synthesize glycogen or glucose. The amino nitrogen derived from the amino acids is detoxified as urea.

Dietary glucose is converted by muscle to lactate prior to glycogen synthesis

It is emphasized that, in the early well-fed state, glucose cannot be used by the liver for glycolysis. Instead, high concentrations of glucose promote hepatic glycogen synthesis. Alternatively, in the presence of insulin, glucose enters the muscle cells, where it undergoes glycolysis to lactate (see Diagram 20.1). Remember that β-oxidation of fatty acids is active and produces an abundance of acetyl CoA, which inhibits muscle pyruvate dehydrogenase. This means that lactate is formed even though conditions are aerobic. The lactate is then transported to the liver, which can convert it to glycogen or glucose.

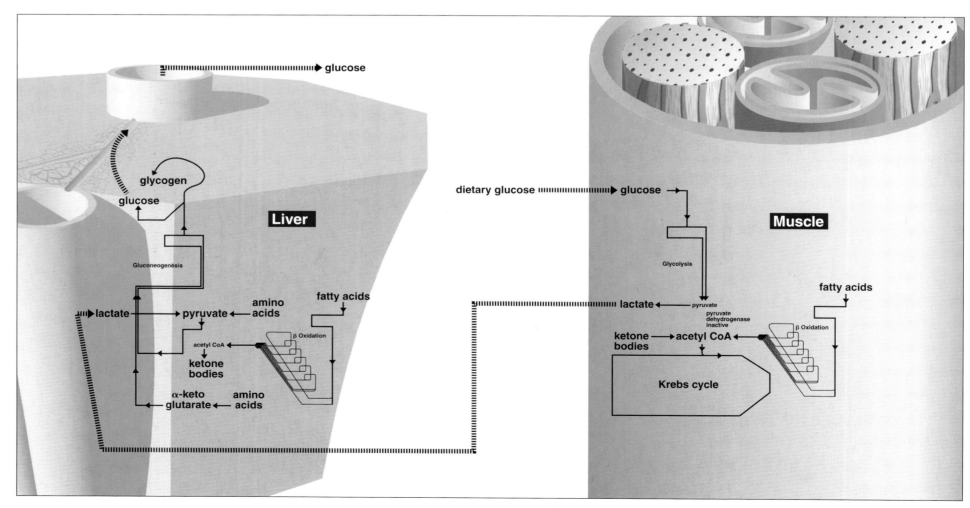

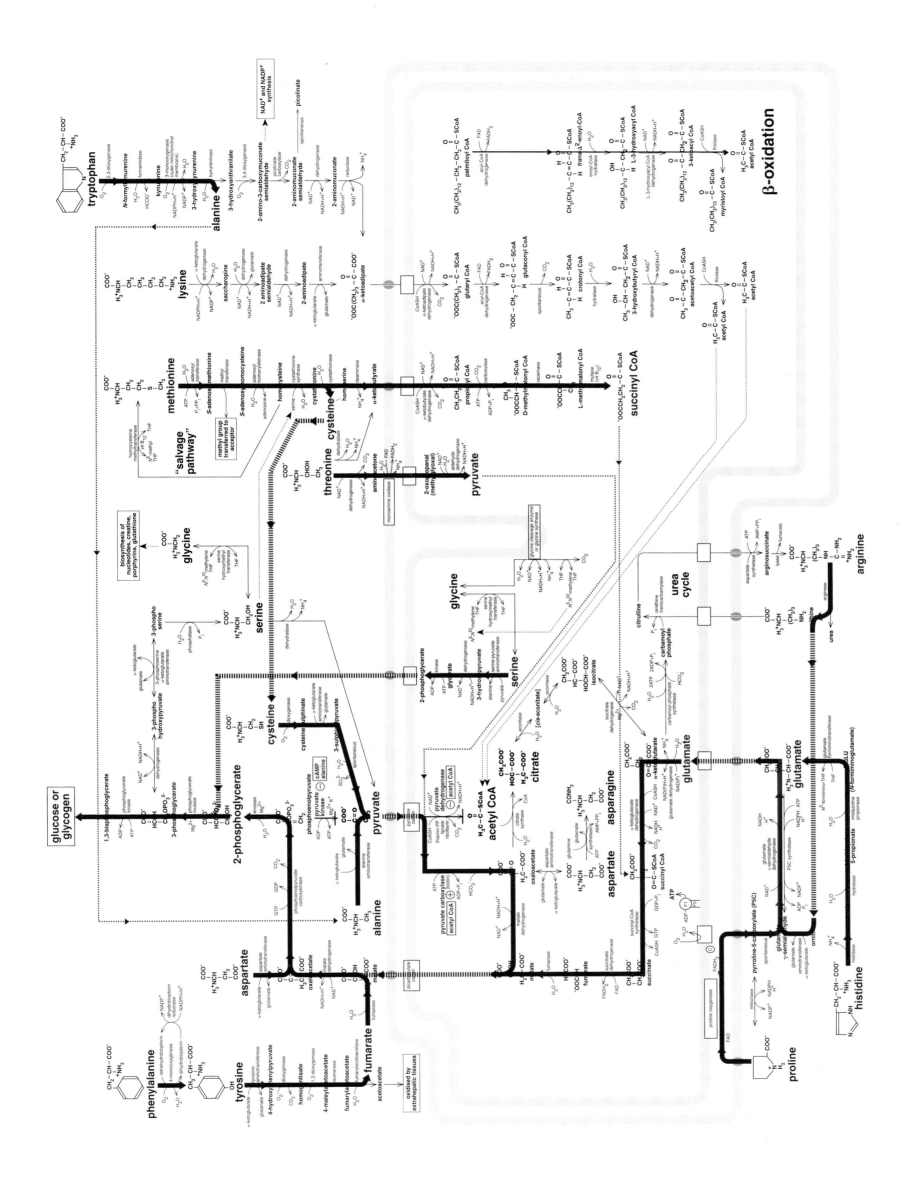

Metabolism of protein to fat

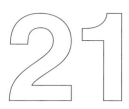

Chart 21 opposite. Metabolism of amino acids to triacylglycerol.

In spite of the exhortation by some popular weight-reducing diets to eat large quantities of protein, it should be remembered that surplus dietary protein **can** be converted to fat. For protein to be converted to fatty acids and triacylglycerols, the essential precursors for fatty acid synthesis, namely a carbon source, **acetyl CoA**, and biosynthetic reducing power as **NADPH+H⁺**, must be formed.

Chart 21: Metabolism of amino acids to triacylglycerol
Metabolism of protein to acetyl CoA

Dietary protein is digested by gastric and intestinal proteolytic enzymes to form amino acids, which are absorbed into the blood and transported to the liver. Here (with the notable exception of the branched-chain amino acids), transamination with α-ketoglutarate produces glutamate and the corresponding α-ketoacids. The amino nitrogen is detoxified in the form of urea.

The carbon skeletons derived from phenylalanine, tyrosine, threonine, glycine, serine, cysteine, alanine, tryptophan, methionine, valine, isoleucine, glutamate, proline, histidine, aspartate and arginine enter the pathways for metabolism to pyruvate as shown in the chart. The pyruvate thus formed enters the mitochondrion and can proceed either via **pyruvate carboxylase** to oxaloacetate, entering the pyruvate / malate cycle (see Chapter 13), or it can be decarboxylated to acetyl CoA by **pyruvate dehydrogenase**.

The ketogenic amino acids (and fragments of the dual, glucogenic / ketogenic amino acids), namely lysine, tryptophan, leucine and isoleucine, are metabolized to acetyl CoA. (**NB:** Although phenylalanine and tyrosine, when degraded, yield acetoacetate, this cannot be metabolized by the liver and so is likely to be exported for use as a respiratory fuel elsewhere (see Chapter 35). Since fatty acid synthesis occurs in the cytosol, acetyl CoA is transported from the mitochondrion to the cytosol by a process known as the **pyruvate / malate cycle** (see Chapter 13). This involves the transport of citrate to the cytosol, where it is cleaved by citrate lyase to form oxaloacetate and **acetyl CoA**. The acetyl CoA is now available for fatty acid synthesis.

Sources of NADPH+H⁺
Pyruvate / malate cycle

In Chapter 20, the metabolism of amino acids to glucose in the starved state was described. Furthermore, it was explained that, following refeeding, there is a transitional period during which the liver remains in gluconeogenic mode, notwithstanding the fact that it now has an abundant supply of glucose for glycolysis. Moreover, lipolysis and β-oxidation of fatty acids continue during this transition period. However, in due course following refeeding, insulin, which is secreted by the pancreas, gains hormonal dominance, β-oxidation ceases, and fatty acid synthesis prevails.

Insulin acts by activating pyruvate dehydrogenase, thus promoting the oxidative decarboxylation of pyruvate to acetyl CoA and providing a carbon source for lipogenesis. Insulin also inhibits transcription of the phosphoenolpyruvate carboxykinase (PEPCK) gene. This leads to decreased PEPCK activity, and malate formed from the amino acid precursors can no longer be metabolized via oxaloacetate to phosphoenolpyruvate. Consequently, gluconeogenesis is inhibited. Malate now follows an alternative route and is oxidatively decarboxylated by the **malic enzyme** to form pyruvate and **NADPH+H⁺**. The pyruvate / malate cycle is described more fully in Chapter 13.

Pentose phosphate pathway

Providing a source of glucose 6-phosphate is available, e.g. from dietary glucose or fructose, the pentose phosphate pathway can generate NADPH+H⁺ for fatty acid synthesis. This process is described in Chapter 12.

Esterification of fatty acids to triacylglycerols

Glyceraldehyde 3-phosphate formed by the pentose phosphate pathway is in equilibrium with dihydroxyacetone phosphate, which is reduced by glycerol 3-phosphate dehydrogenase to form glycerol 3-phosphate. This can be used to esterify fatty acids, as described in Chapter 32.

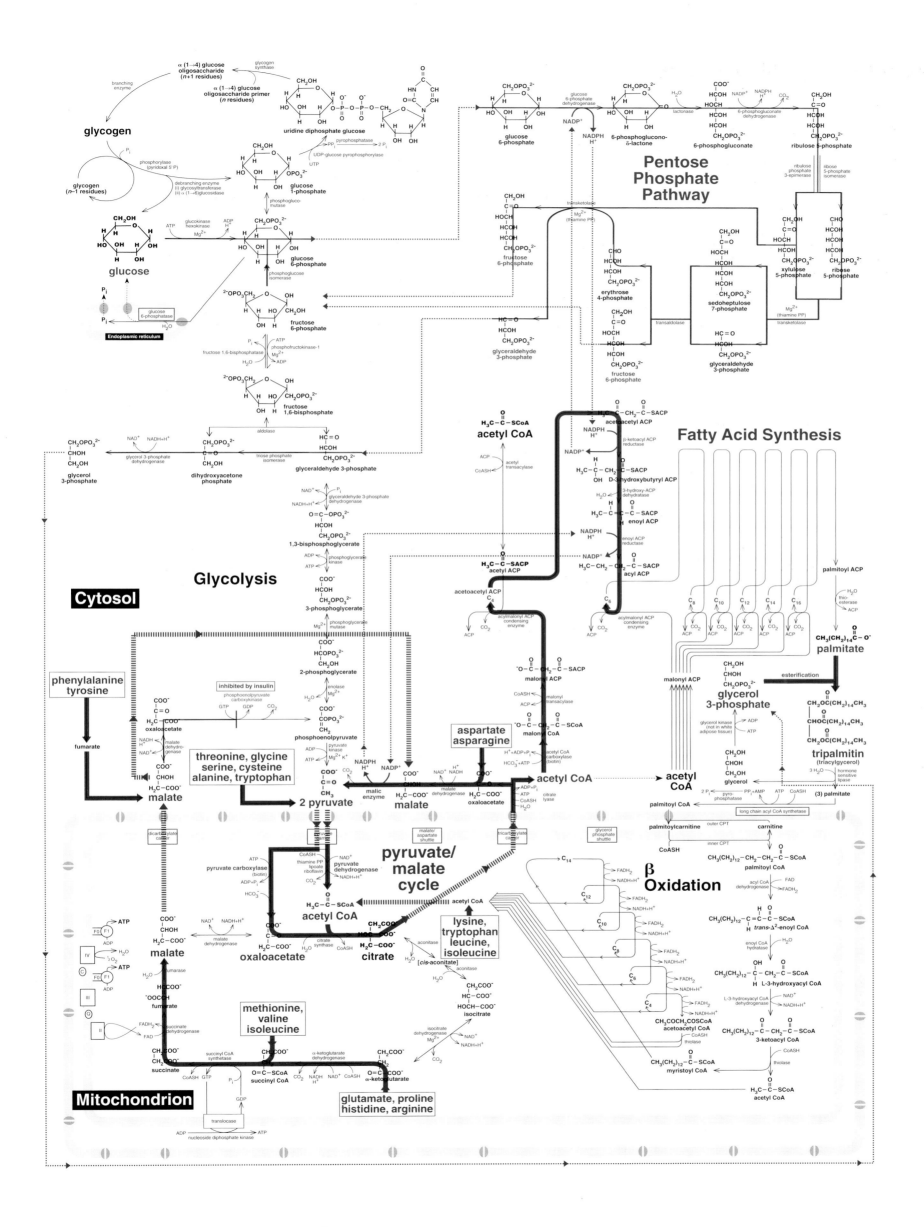

Disorders of amino acid metabolism

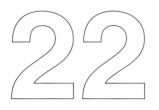

There is a very large body of literature on these rare inborn errors of metabolism which has often contributed to our understanding of normal metabolic processes. A few examples are listed below and/or are indicated on the charts.

Phenylketonuria

This is an autosomal recessive disorder resulting from deficiency of **phenylalanine monooxygenase** activity. Whereas the monooxygenase is usually directly involved, in 3% of cases the disorder is due to impaired synthesis of its coenzyme, **tetrahydrobiopterin**. Because phenylalanine cannot be metabolized to tyrosine, it accumulates and is transaminated to the 'phenylketone', phenylpyruvate.

Chart 22 opposite. Disorders of amino acid metabolism.

Albinism

Tyrosine is metabolized by tyrosinase in melanocytes to form the pigment, melanin. Deficiency of tyrosinase results in albinism.

Alkaptonuria

This autosomal recessive condition is due to deficiency of **homogentisate 1,2-dioxygenase**. Homogentisate accumulates and is excreted in the urine where, under alkaline conditions, it can undergo oxidation and polymerization to form the black pigment, alkapton.

Histidinaemia

This is an autosomal recessive disorder in which deficiency of **histidase** causes an accumulation of histidine.

Maple syrup urine disease

In this autosomal recessive disorder, deficiency of the **branched-chain, α-ketoacid dehydrogenase** complex causes accumulation of the branched-chain amino acids isoleucine, valine and leucine, and their corresponding α-ketoacids. These compounds smell like maple syrup, hence the name of this condition.

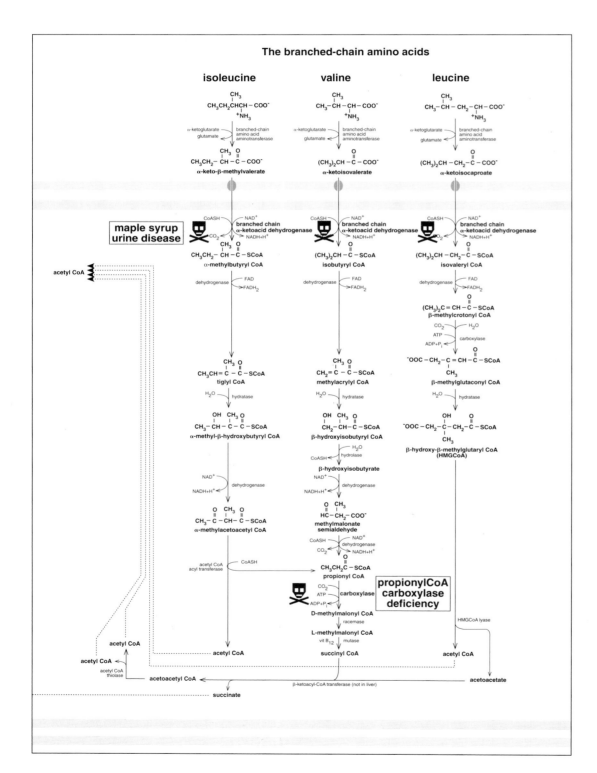

Diagram 22.1. Disorders of branched amino acid metabolism.

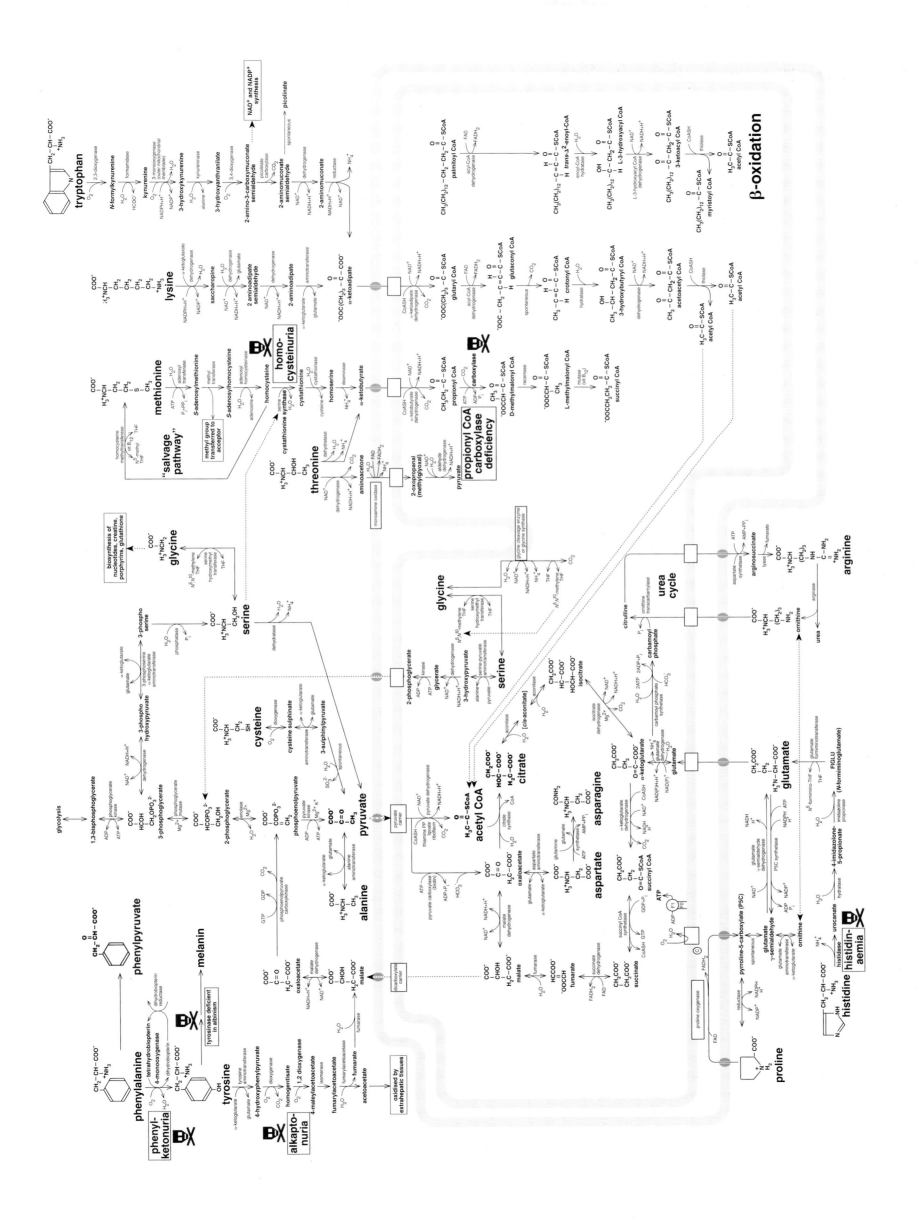

Amino acid metabolism, folate metabolism, and the '1-carbon pool', part I: purine biosynthesis

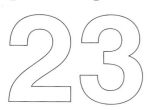

Chart 23 opposite. Purine biosynthesis.

The '1-carbon pool'

This term describes the 1-carbon residues associated with *S*-adenosylmethionine and **folate** which are available for metabolic reactions.

S-Adenosylmethionine (SAM)

SAM, which is formed from methionine, is the major donor of methyl groups for biosynthetic reactions. It can, for example, methylate noradrenaline to form adrenaline, as shown in the chart opposite. Other important reactions involving SAM include the methylation of phosphatidylethanolamine to phosphatidylcholine, and the formation of creatine.

The folate '1-carbon' units

The vitamin folate is reduced in two stages by dihydrofolate reductase to produce the active form, **tetrahydrofolate (THF)**. THF is a versatile carrier of 1-carbon units in the following oxidation states: methyl, methylene, methenyl, and formyl. These THF compounds, which are interconvertible, together with SAM, comprise what is known as the '1-carbon' pool.

Amino acids and the '1-carbon' pool

Serine is converted to **glycine**, in a reaction catalysed by **serine hydroxymethyl transferase**, with the transfer of a methyl group to the THF so as to form N^5, N^{10}-methylene THF. This reaction is particularly important in the thymidylate synthase reaction described in Chapter 24. Oxidation of glycine in mitochondria by the glycine cleavage enzyme also produces N^5, N^{10}-methylene THF (see Chapter 19).

Tryptophan is oxidized to *N*-formylkynurenine which, in the presence of formamidase, yields kynurenine and the toxic product **formate**. THF accepts the formate, producing N^{10}-**formyl THF**.

Methionine, as mentioned above, is the precursor of SAM which, following transfer of the methyl group, forms homocysteine. Methionine can be regenerated from homocysteine by methylation using N^5-methyl THF in a salvage pathway. **NB:** This reaction, catalysed by homocysteine methyltransferase, requires **vitamin B$_{12}$**, and lack of this vitamin can lead to folate being caught in the 'methyl–folate' trap (see below).

Amino acid metabolism and purine synthesis

Glycine contributes the C-4, C-5, and N-7 atoms to the purine ring in a reaction catalysed by glycinamide ribonucleotide (GAR) synthetase (see Chart 23).

Aspartate is an important donor of nitrogen atoms during purine biosynthesis, contributing the N-1 atom to the purine ring, and the $-NH_2$ group in the adenylosuccinate synthetase reaction of the pathway which forms AMP from inosine monophosphate (IMP) (see Diagram 23.1).

Glutamine plays a very important role in nucleotide metabolism. It donates the nitrogen atoms which form N-9 and N-3 of the purine ring. It also participates in the amination of xanthine monophosphate (XMP) to form guanosine monophosphate (GMP) (Diagram 23.1).

Biosynthesis of purines

Purine nucleotides can be synthesized *de novo*. They can also be reclaimed from existing nucleosides by the so-called 'salvage pathway' (see Chapter 24). The *de novo* pathway needs '1-carbon' units from the folate pool, and several amino acids as detailed below.

De novo pathway for purine biosynthesis

The pathway starts with **ribose 5-phosphate** formed by the pentose phosphate pathway (see Chart 23). This is activated to form **phosphoribosyl pyrophosphate (PRPP)**. A total of 11 reactions is needed to form **IMP** (inosine monophosphate or inosinic acid), which is the precursor of the adenine- and guanine-containing nucleotides. The important roles of glutamine and aspartate as amino donors are emphasized. A total of three glutamine molecules and one aspartate molecule is needed for the synthesis of GMP. Similarly, a total of two glutamine and two aspartate molecules is needed for AMP synthesis. A molecule of glycine is needed in each case.

The *de novo* pathway is controlled by feedback inhibition of PRPP amidotransferase by AMP and GMP. In primary gout this feedback control is impaired, causing increased production of purines resulting in the increased formation of their sparingly soluble excretory product, urate.

Vitamin B$_{12}$ and the 'methyl–folate trap'

Vitamin B$_{12}$, or more precisely its methyl cobalamin derivative, is an essential coenzyme for the transfer of methyl groups in the **methionine salvage pathway** (see Chart 23). Accordingly, in B$_{12}$ deficiency, THF cannot be released and remains trapped as N^5-methyl THF. Eventually, according to the hypothesis, all the body's folate becomes trapped in the N^5-methyl THF form, and so folate deficiency develops secondary to B$_{12}$ deficiency. Because blood cells turn over rapidly, they need nucleotides for nucleic acid synthesis and are vulnerable to folate deficiency, which causes megaloblastic anaemia.

The methyl–folate trap hypothesis explains the observation that, although the haematological symptoms of B$_{12}$ deficiency respond to folate treatment, the neurological degeneration progresses. Remember that the other enzyme for which B$_{12}$ is a coenzyme is methylmalonyl CoA mutase (see Chapters 18 and 19). Accumulation of methylmalonyl CoA may interfere with the biosynthesis of lipids needed for the myelin sheath.

Diagram 23.1.

Conversion of IMP to ATP. IMP reacts with aspartate in the presence of GTP to form adenylosuccinate, which is cleaved to form fumarate and AMP. The AMP can be phosphorylated to ADP, which undergoes oxidative phosphorylation to form ATP.

Conversion of IMP to GTP. IMP is oxidized to xanthine monophosphate (XMP), which is aminated to form GMP, which is phosphorylated to form GDP. GDP is phosphorylated by ATP in a reaction catalysed by nucleoside diphosphate kinase. Alternatively, when the Krebs cycle is active, GTP is formed from GDP by succinyl CoA synthetase.

Formation of dATP (deoxyadenosine triphosphate) and dGTP (deoxyguanosine triphosphate). The deoxyribonucleotides dATP and dGTP are formed by first reducing ADP and GDP to dADP and dGDP in the presence of ribonucleotide reductase. These are subsequently phosphorylated to form dATP and dGTP, which can be used for the synthesis of DNA.

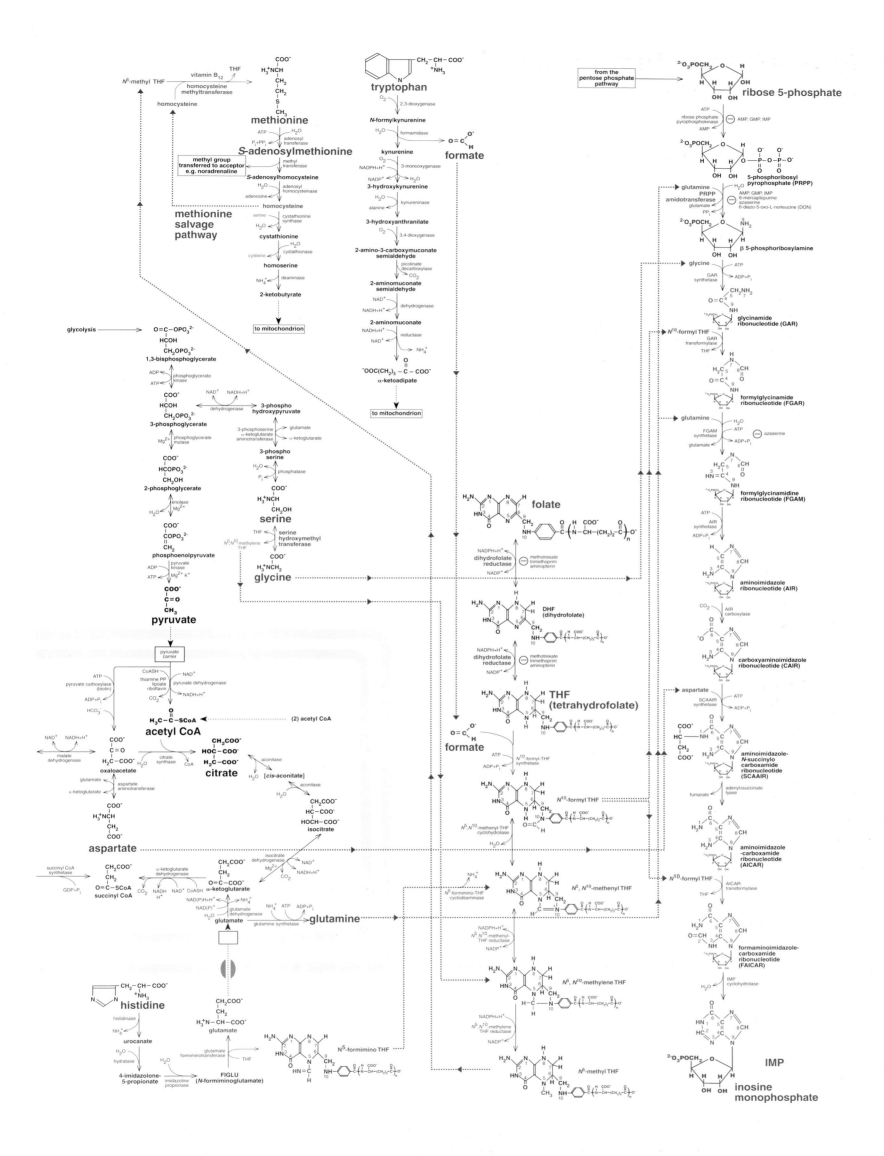

Amino acid metabolism, folate metabolism, and the '1-carbon pool', part II: pyrimidine biosynthesis

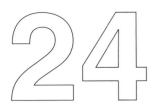

Chart 24 opposite. Biosynthesis of pyrimidines.

Amino acid metabolism and pyrimidine biosynthesis

The pyrimidine ring is derived from glutamine, aspartate and bicarbonate. The first reaction occurs in the cytosol and produces **carbamoyl phosphate** from bicarbonate, glutamine and two molecules of ATP. This is similar to the mitochondrial reaction involved in the urea cycle, which differs in that it forms carbamoyl phosphate from bicarbonate and NH_4^+ ions. The rest of the pyrimidine ring is donated by aspartate and, after ring closure and oxidation, **orotate** is formed. It is at this stage that **phosphoribosyl pyrophosphate (PRPP)** is added to yield **orotidine monophosphate (OMP)** which, following decarboxylation, produces **uridine monophosphate (UMP)**, which is the common precursor of the pyrimidine-containing nucleotides.

Conversion of UMP to UTP and CTP

UMP is phosphorylated by a specific UMP kinase to form uridine diphosphate (UDP), which in turn is phosphorylated by the non-specific nucleoside diphosphate kinase to yield **uridine triphosphate (UTP)**. When UTP is aminated, **cytidine triphosphate (CTP)** is formed.

Formation of deoxycytidine triphosphate (dCTP) and deoxythymidine triphosphate (dTTP)

dCTP is formed from CDP by ribonucleotide reductase, as described for the production of the purine-containing deoxyribonucleotides in Chapter 23.

The pathway for the formation of dTTP is quite distinct from that used to produce dATP, dGTP and dCTP. The pathway starts with dCDP, which is dephosphorylated and deaminated to yield **deoxyuridine monophosphate (dUMP)**. This is methylated by N^5,N^{10}-**methylene THF** which is oxidized to **dihydrofolate (DHF)** in the reaction catalysed by **thymidylate synthase**, and **deoxythymidine monophosphate (dTMP)** is formed. The dTMP is now phosphorylated by dTMP kinase and nucleoside diphosphate kinase to produce dTTP.

Let us return to the DHF, which is formed by the thymidylate synthase reaction. This is reduced by **dihydrofolate reductase**, which regenerates **tetrahydrofolate (THF)**. The cycle is completed when this THF participates in the serine hydroxymethyltransferase reaction which produces glycine and N^5,N^{10}-methylene THF, which is now available once more for the thymidylate synthase reaction.

Cancer chemotherapy

Because rapidly dividing cancer cells have a great demand for DNA synthesis, much attention has been directed at the pathways for nucleotide synthesis as the target for chemotherapeutic intervention. These drugs are classified by pharmacologists as 'antimetabolites' and fall into the following categories: glutamine antagonists, folate antagonists, antipyrimidines and antipurines.

Glutamine antagonists

The importance of glutamine for the biosynthesis of purines and pyrimidines has been emphasized already. Azaserine and diazo-oxo-norleucine (DON) irreversibly inhibit the enzymes involved in the glutamine-utilizing reactions (see Chart 23), and reduce the supply of DNA available to cancer cells.

Folate antagonists

Methotrexate, which is a close structural analogue of folate, inhibits DHF reductase. This prevents the reduction of DHF to THF, as shown in the chart opposite. Consequently, in the absence of THF, serine hydroxymethyltransferase is unable to generate the N^5,N^{10}-methylene-THF needed by thymidylate synthase for dTMP production.

methotrexate

The clinical benefit to patients treated with high doses of methotrexate is improved by the use of folinic acid, N^5-formyl THF (also known as leucovorin), which 'rescues' normal cells from the toxic effects of methotrexate.

Antipyrimidines

Fluorouracil inhibits thymidylate synthase and thus prevents the conversion of dUMP to dTMP.

Antipurines

Mercaptopurine inhibits purine biosynthesis at several stages. It inhibits PRPP-amidotransferase (see Chart 23), IMP dehydrogenase and adenylosuccinate synthetase (see Diagram 23.1).

Salvage pathways for the recycling of purines and pyrimidines

When nucleic acids and nucleotides are degraded, the free purine and pyrimidine bases are formed. These can be recycled by 'salvage pathways' which require much less ATP compared with the energy-intensive *de novo* pathways. The salvage pathways require specific **phosphoribosyl transferases (PRTs)** whose functions are analogous to that of **orotate PRT** (see chart opposite).

AMP salvage

$$\text{adenine } + \text{ PRPP } \xrightarrow{\text{adenine PRT}} \text{AMP } + \text{ PP}_i$$

IMP and GMP salvage

Both hypoxanthine and guanine can be used as substrates by the enzyme involved:

$$\text{hypoxanthine } + \text{ PRPP } \xrightarrow{\qquad} \text{IMP } + \text{ PP}_i$$
$$\xrightarrow{\text{hypoxanthine–guanine PRT}}$$
$$\text{guanine } + \text{ PRPP } \xrightarrow{\qquad} \text{GMP } + \text{ PP}_i$$

UMP and TMP salvage

$$\text{uracil } + \text{ PRPP } \xrightarrow{\qquad} \text{UMP } + \text{ PP}_i$$
$$\xrightarrow{\text{uracil–thymine PRT}}$$
$$\text{thymine } + \text{ PRPP } \xrightarrow{\qquad} \text{TMP } + \text{ PP}_i$$

NB: Uracil-thymine PRT cannot use cytosine as a substrate.

Lesch–Nyhan syndrome

This is an extremely rare disorder caused by almost total deficiency of hypoxanthine-guanine PRT. In this condition, which is characterized by severe self-mutilation, the salvage pathway is inactive. Consequently, the free purines hypoxanthine and guanine, are instead oxidized by xanthine oxidase to urate.

The antiviral drug AZT (azidothymidine)

AZT is an analogue of thymidine which can be phosphorylated to form the nucleotide triphosphate, azidothymidine triphosphate (AZTTP).

AZTTP inhibits the viral DNA-polymerase which is an RNA-dependent polymerase. The host cell's DNA-dependent polymerase is relatively insensitive to inhibition by AZTTP.

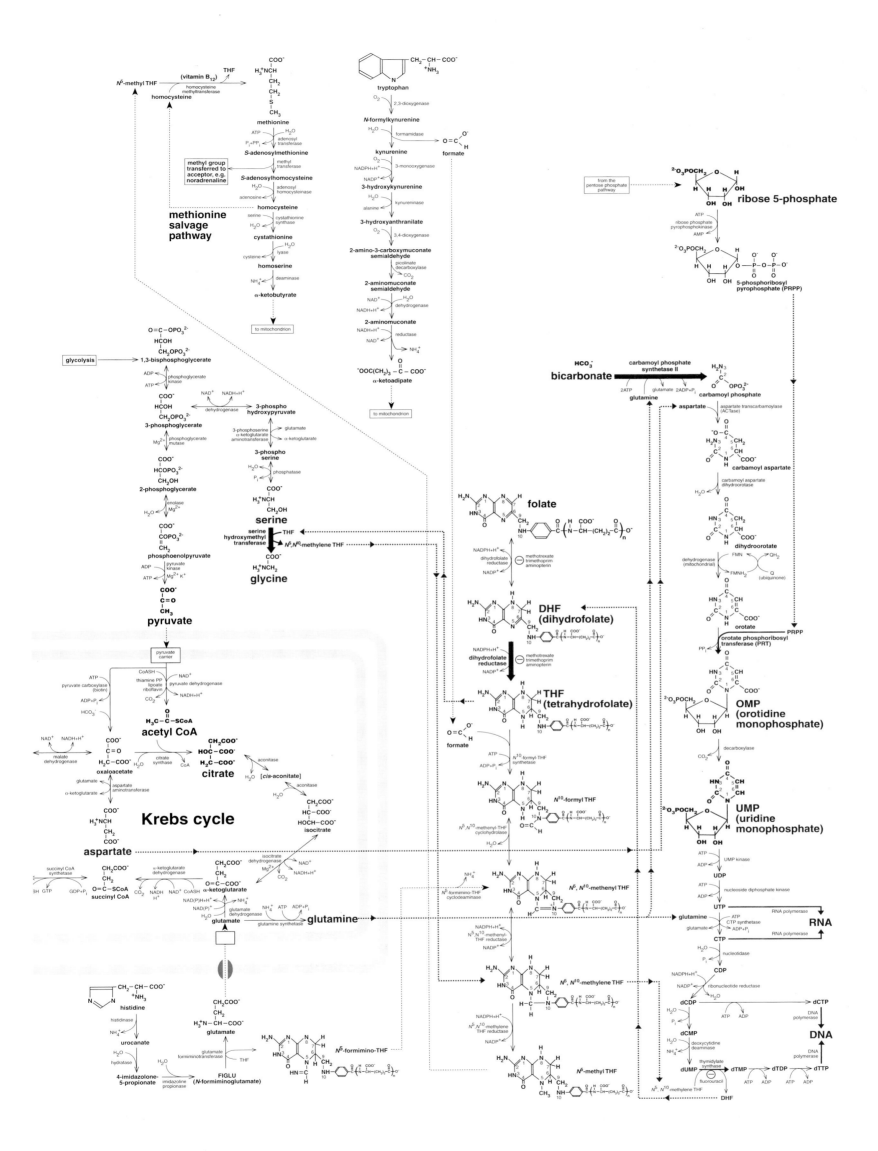

Glycogen metabolism, part I

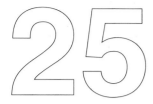

The different roles of glycogen in liver and muscle

Although both liver and muscle store glycogen, there are major differences between the two in the way that glycogen metabolism is deployed and controlled. The liver exports glucose derived from glycogen for use by other tissues. In skeletal muscle, the glucose is particularly important as a fuel which is immediately available during periods of extreme activity, such as in the adrenaline-driven 'flight or fight' response.

The metabolic demands made on glycogen metabolism

The simplistic approach to glycogen metabolism is to consider glycogen synthesis in the well-fed state, followed by glycogen breakdown during fasting or 'flight or fight', followed by glycogen synthesis in the well-fed state to complete the cycle. However, nature does not order periods of feeding, fasting and flight with carefully planned transition periods in between. Indeed, in nature, animals are very vulnerable to attack by a predator when they are feeding. The prey's muscles must then respond to the crisis by instantly diverting the flux of glucose metabolites from the feeding state of glycogen **synthesis** to glycogen **breakdown** for anaerobic glycolysis. Furthermore, this instantaneous metabolic U-turn must be achieved in spite of the lingering presence of insulin secreted during feeding, which tends to promote glycogen synthesis. Next, after a strenuous chase, the prey (assuming it has survived) must quickly replenish its glycogen reserves for the next emergency, whether food is available or not. Moreover, this must be done without excessively draining blood glucose concentrations and causing hypoglycaemia. Not surprisingly, the complicated physiological demands made on glycogen metabolism are matched by a complicated regulatory mechanism. The details of this mechanism are still not fully understood, but it involves an **amplification cascade** which dramatically enhances the effects of the hormones, which initiate this series of reactions (see Chapter 26).

Glycogen metabolism: an overview

Liver and muscle share some general features during the processes of glycogen synthesis from glucose 1-phosphate, and glycogenolysis back to glucose 1-phosphate. These are summarized as follows.

Glycogenesis

Glucose 1-phosphate reacts with **uridine triphosphate (UTP)** to form **uridine diphosphate glucose (UDP-glucose)**. This is an activated form of glucose used for glycogen synthesis. A **primer** in the form of an $\alpha(1\rightarrow4)$ glucose oligosaccharide attached to the protein glycogenin is also needed (Chart 25.2). The glucosyl group from UDP-glucose is added to the polysaccharide chain by **glycogen synthase** provided it consists of four or more glucose residues. Once the chain contains 11 or more residues, the **branching enzyme** becomes involved. The branching enzyme forms the many branches of glycogen by severing a string of seven residues from the growing chain and rejoining it by an $\alpha(1\rightarrow6)$ linkage to an interior point at least four residues from an existing branch.

Glycogenolysis

The enzyme controlling glycogenolysis is **phosphorylase**. It requires pyridoxal phosphate and inorganic phosphate and exists in both active and inactive forms. Phosphorylase progressively nibbles its way along the chain of $\alpha(1\rightarrow4)$ glucose molecules, releasing molecules of **glucose 1-phosphate**. Its progress is obstructed when it reaches a stage on the chain four glucose residues away from a branch point. Another enzyme, **glycosyl transferase**, rescues the situation by transferring the terminal three (of these four) glucose molecules to the end of another chain so that phosphorylase activity can continue. The remaining glucose molecule, which now forms an $\alpha(1\rightarrow6)$ linked stump at the branching point, is removed as free glucose by $\alpha(1\rightarrow6)$ **glucosidase**.

The glucose 1-phosphate formed by phosphorylase is converted to glucose 6-phosphate by phosphoglucomutase.

Glycogen metabolism in liver

The liver stores glycogen as a reserve fuel for periods of fasting or 'fight or flight'. Liver does not usually use the glycogen-derived glucose itself for energy : instead it is exported for use by the brain, red blood cells and, in a crisis, by muscle.

Glycogenolysis in liver

Glycogenolysis (Chart 25.1) is stimulated by glucagon in response to fasting, and by adrenaline for 'fight and flight'. Both of these hormones stimulate the **glycogenolysis cascade** (Diagram 26.1) to produce glucose 6-phosphate. Liver (unlike muscle) has glucose 6-phosphatase, which enables mobilization of glucose into the blood.

Note that, in liver (in contrast to muscle), cyclic AMP-mediated phosphorylation **inhibits** glycolysis and stimulates hepatic gluconeogenesis (see Chapter 29). In the physiological context this means that during fasting, when glucagon is present, both glycogenolysis and gluconeogenesis will be active.

Glycogen synthesis in liver
From dietary carbohydrate

Glycogen synthesis (see Chart 25.2) occurs in the well-fed state when glucose arrives at the liver in very high concentrations. The liver glucose transporter, Glu T2, works independently of insulin, and glucose enters the cell and is phosphorylated by glucokinase to glucose 6-phosphate. It might appear at first glance that, in theory, glucose 6-phosphate could enter glycolysis. However, in the well-fed state phosphofructokinase-1 is inhibited (see Chapter 29). Glucose 6-phosphate could also enter the pentose phosphate pathway, and probably does so to generate $NADPH+H^+$ for fatty acid synthesis. Nevertheless, replenishment of the glycogen reserves is very important and in Chart 25.2 this is shown in the early fed state as having priority over fatty acid synthesis.

From lactate

During anaerobic glycolysis, lactate produced by the muscles accumulates in the blood pending aerobic recovery and is used for gluconeogenesis and glycogen synthesis by the liver (see Chapter 8). In the early well-fed state after a period of fasting, lactate is also produced by muscle for glycogen synthesis, even though conditions are aerobic. This is because, after refeeding, the high ratio of acetyl CoA / CoA caused by the lingering activity of β-oxidation results in pyruvate dehydrogenase remaining inhibited under these conditions (see Chapter 20). Consequently, when glucose is metabolized in muscle by the glycolytic pathway, the pyruvate formed is reduced to lactate, which is transported to the liver for use as a gluconeogenic substrate prior to glycogen synthesis.

Chart 25.1. Glycogenolysis in liver.

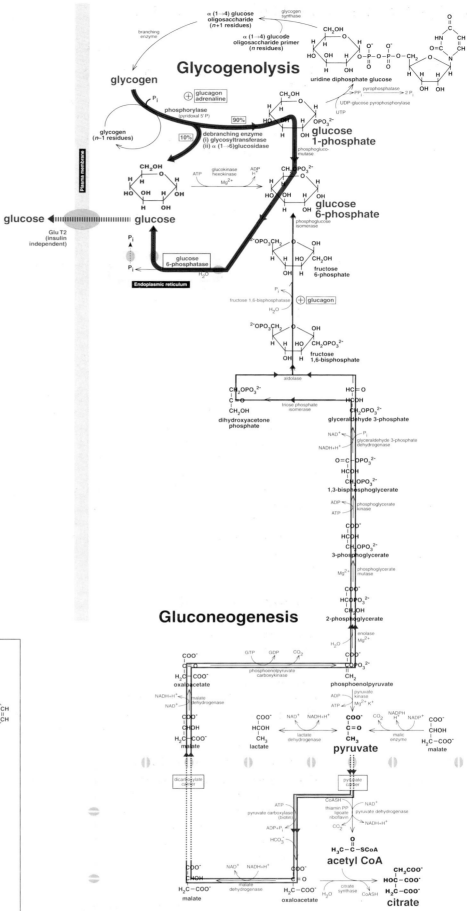

Chart 25.2. Glycogenesis in liver.

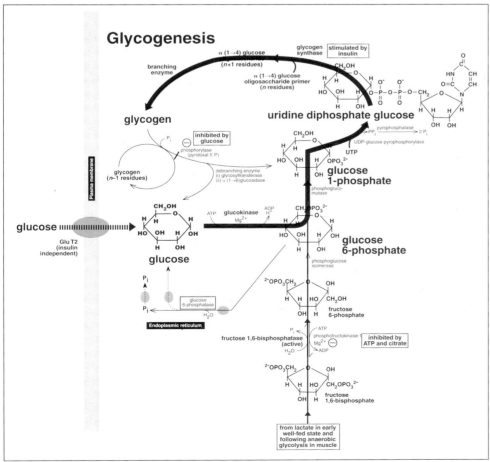

Glycogen metabolism, part II

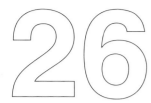

Glycogen metabolism in muscle
In muscle, the main function of glycogen is to serve as a reserve of respiratory fuel by rapidly providing glucose during periods of extremely vigorous muscle contraction, such as occur in moments of danger, i.e. in the 'fight or flight response'.

Glycogenolysis in skeletal muscle
Glycogenolysis in muscle (Chart 26.1) is stimulated by adrenaline via the amplification cascade shown in Diagram 26.1. **Phosphorylase** produces **glucose 1-phosphate**, which is converted into **glucose 6-phosphate**. Because muscle lacks glucose 6-phosphatase, glucose 6-phosphate is totally committed to glycolysis for ATP production. Also, since muscle hexokinase has a very low K_m for glucose (0.1 mmol/l), it has a very high affinity for glucose and will readily phosphorylate the 10% of glucose units liberated from glycogen by the debranching enzyme (α (1→6) glucosidase) as free glucose, thus ensuring its use by glycolysis. It should be remembered that adrenaline increases the cyclic AMP concentration, which not only stimulates glycogenolysis but **in muscle** also stimulates glycolysis (see Chapter 29).

Glycogen synthesis in skeletal muscle
In the well-fed state, in resting muscle, insulin is available to facilitate glucose transport into the muscle cell using the Glu T4 transporter (see Chart 26.2). Remember that, in the well-fed state, phosphofructokinase is inhibited (see Chapter 29) and so glucose 6-phosphate will be used for glycogen synthesis. It should be noted that glycogen synthesis and glycogenolysis are regulated in a reciprocal way (Diagram 26.1).

The glycogenolysis cascade
Diagram 26.1 shows how the original signal provided by a single molecule of adrenaline is amplified during the course of a cascade of reactions which activate a large number of phosphorylase molecules, ensuring the rapid mobilization of glycogen as follows:

1 A molecule of adrenaline stimulates adenyl cyclase to form several molecules of **cyclic AMP**.

2 Each molecule of cyclic AMP dissociates an inactive tetramer to free two catalytically active monomers of **cyclic AMP-dependent protein kinase** (also known as **protein kinase A**) from their regulatory monomers. **NB**: This gives a relatively modest amplification factor of two.

3 Each active molecule of cyclic AMP-dependent protein kinase phosphorylates and activates several molecules of **phosphorylase kinase**.

At this point, reciprocal regulation of glycogen synthesis and breakdown occurs. First, let us continue with glycogenolysis before concluding with the inactivation of glycogen synthesis.

4 One molecule of phosphorylase kinase phosphorylates several inactive molecules of **phosphorylase b** to give the active form, **phosphorylase a**, and so glycogen breakdown can now proceed.

Inactivation of glycogen synthesis
To maximize glycogen breakdown, synthesis is reciprocally inactivated by phosphorylase kinase, which is one of several protein kinases, including cyclic AMP-dependent protein kinase, which can phosphorylate **glycogen synthase a** to give its low activity **synthase b** form (see Diagram 26.1).

Reference
Cohen P., Signal integration at the level of protein kinases, protein phosphatases and their substrates. *TIBS* **17**, 408–413, 1992.

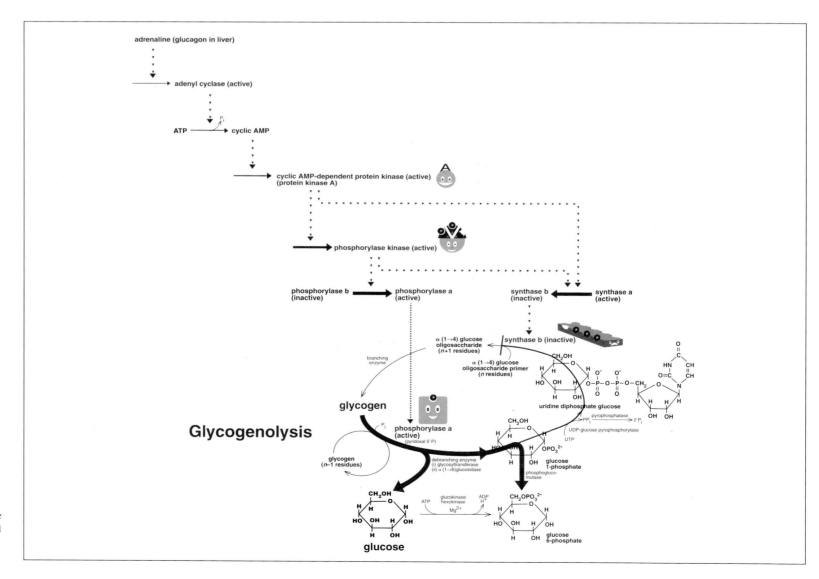

Diagram 26.1. Activation of the glycogenolysis cascade is linked to the inactivation of glycogen synthesis

Chart 26.1. Glycogenolysis in muscle.

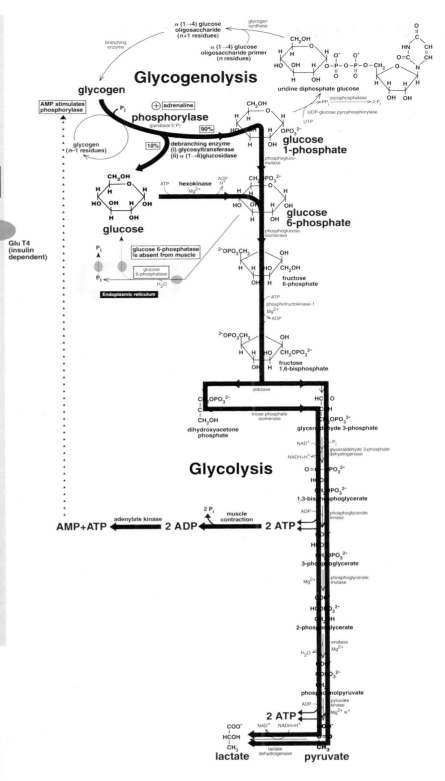

Chart 26.2. Glycogenesis in muscle.

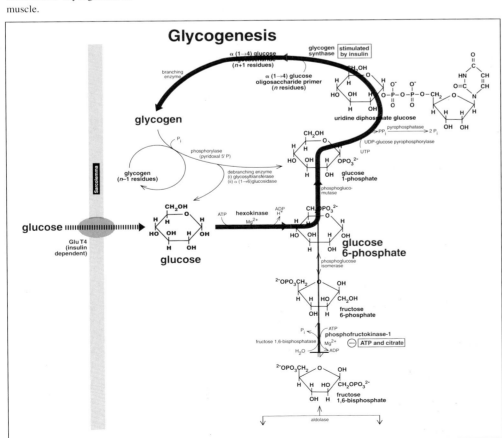

Glycogen metabolism, part III: regulation of glycogen breakdown

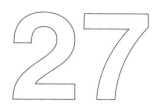

27

Chart 27 opposite. Regulation of glycogenolysis.

Hormonal control: the role of adrenaline and glucagon in the regulation of glycogenolysis

In liver, glycogenolysis is stimulated by both glucagon and adrenaline, whereas in muscle only adrenaline is effective. In a crisis, when mobilization of glycogen is stimulated by adrenaline, the response must happen **immediately!** This occurs through the remarkable amplification cascade described earlier (see Chapter 26), in which cyclic AMP plays an important role. In this way, small, nanomolar concentrations of adrenaline can rapidly mobilize a vast number of glucose residues for use as respiratory fuel.

*NB : The regulation of glycogen metabolism, which is complex, is still the subject of extensive research and full details are beyond the scope of this book. **The descriptions provided here and in the next chapter are based on current knowledge, largely relating to the regulation of glycogen metabolism in skeletal muscle.** Whereas many details of the mechanisms may be common to both liver and muscle, there are several differences stemming from the different functions of the two tissues, e.g. whereas both liver and muscle are responsive to adrenaline (albeit through different mechanisms), only liver has receptors for glucagon.*

Chart 27: Regulation of glycogenolysis
Formation of cyclic AMP
When adrenaline docks with its receptor in muscle, the signal is transduced through the G protein, **adenyl cyclase** is activated, and ATP is converted to **cyclic AMP,** which activates **cyclic AMP-dependent protein kinase**.

Cyclic AMP-dependent protein kinase (also known as protein kinase A)
When inactive, cyclic AMP-dependent protein kinase exists as part of a tetramer consisting of two catalytic subunits and two regulatory (R) subunits (see Diagram 27.1). When cyclic AMP is present, it binds to the two regulatory units and liberates the two active catalytic subunits.

NB : *These active monomers of cyclic AMP-dependent protein kinase (and their metabolic opponents, the protein phosphatases, described more fully in the next chapter) play a key role in regulating not only glycogen metabolism, but also many other pathways of intermediary metabolism (see Chapters 29, 31, 32).*

Returning to glycogen metabolism: cyclic AMP-dependent protein kinase plays a major role in both **activating** glycogenolysis and concurrently enhancing this function by **inhibiting** glycogen synthesis.

Roles of cyclic AMP-dependent protein kinase in regulating glycogenolysis
Cyclic AMP-dependent protein kinase phosphorylates several enzymes involved in glycogen metabolism, and these covalent modifications persist until the enzymes are dephosphorylated by protein phosphatases (see Chapter 28). The effects of cyclic AMP-dependent protein kinase, shown in the chart opposite, are:

1 Activation of phosphorylase kinase. Cyclic AMP-dependent protein kinase phosphorylates phosphorylase kinase to yield the active form. However, full activity requires Ca^{2+} ions, which are released into the sarcoplasm when muscle is contracting (or following α-adrenergic stimulation of liver). The fully activated phosphorylase kinase now has a double action: not only does it activate phosphorylase by forming **phosphorylase a** (see Chart 27), but it also participates in phosphorylating (and thus inactivating) glycogen synthase.

2 Inactivation of protein phosphatase-1. Protein phosphatase-1 (see Chapter 28) plays a major role in switching off glycogenolysis by converting phosphorylase a (the active form) to the inactive phosphorylase b. Clearly this must be stopped. Accordingly, protein phosphatase-1 is inactivated by two assassins in the forms of cyclic AMP-dependent protein kinase and the **protein phosphatase inhibitor** (see last paragraph below). The first attack is by cyclic AMP-dependent protein kinase, which phosphorylates site 2 of the regulatory subunit of the protein phosphatase–1G complex. The conse-

quence of this covalent modification is that protein phosphatase-1 dissociates from its sanctuary in the complex. The free protein phosphatase-1 is relatively inactive. Moreover, it is now unprotected and vulnerable to a second attack by the protein phosphatase inhibitor, which diffuses into action and delivers the *coup de grâce*.

So, finally, with the counterproductive interference by protein phosphatase-1 activity well and truly suppressed, phosphorylase a activity prevails unchallenged and glycogen breakdown can now take place.

3 Activation of the protein phosphatase inhibitor-1. The conspiracy between cyclic AMP-dependent protein kinase and the protein phosphatase inhibitor-1 is initiated when the latter is phosphorylated to its active form by the former. The active inhibitor can now join cyclic AMP-dependent protein kinase in the vendetta against protein phosphatase, as described in the previous paragraph.

Phosphorylase kinase
This is a very large 1300 kDa protein and is a hexadecamer of four subunits (see Diagram 27.2). Each subunit consists of an α, β, γ and δ subunits; the native protein thus comprising $\alpha_4\beta_4\gamma_4\delta_4$. The catalytic site is on the γ subunit.

The α and β subunits are phosphorylated during modification from the inactive b form to the active phosphorylase kinase a. Although phosphorylation of the α subunit causes some stimulation of activity, it is the subsequent rapid phosphorylation of the β subunit which is the major activator of phosphorylase kinase activity. The δ subunit is composed of calmodulin, which has four regulatory binding sites with different affinities for calcium. They can bind calcium even at concentrations as low as 0.1 μmol/l, such as occur in resting muscle. However, they are fully occupied and maximally stimulated following the 100-fold increase in calcium concentration of up to 10 μmol/l that occurs during exercise.

Phosphorylase kinase a is inhibited when it is dephosphorylated by **protein phosphatase-1**, which removes phosphate from the β subunit, and by **protein phosphatase-2A**, which demodifies the α subunit (see Chart 28).

Properties of glycogen phosphorylase
Phosphorylase b is a dimer of two identical 97 kDa proteins which are associated with glycogen, and which can be phosphorylated at the serine residue at N-14 by phosphorylase kinase to form **phosphorylase a**. The latter is a tetramer formed by dimerization of phosphorylase b. (For simplicity, the monomer is shown in the chart).

In resting muscle, phosphorylase b is in the inactive T form; in contracting muscle it is in the active R form. During exercise, ATP is converted to AMP. The increase in AMP concentration stimulates phosphorylase b by forming the R form which decreases its K_m for phosphate. Conversely, ATP and glucose 6-phosphate counter the effect of AMP so that in the resting state, as the concentrations of the former recover, phosphorylase b is converted back to the inactive T form.

Phosphorylase a is not dependent on AMP for activity, provided the concentration of P_i is sufficiently increased, as happens during muscle contraction. It is formed by the action of phosphorylase kinase, as described above and undergoes a conformational change from the T form to the active R form.

Inactivation of phosphorylase a is by demodification by protein phosphatase-1 (see Chart 28).

Protein phosphatase inhibitor-1
The inhibitor-1 is an 18.7 kDa protein which is modified to its active form by phosphorylation of a threonine residue in a reaction catalysed by cyclic AMP-dependent protein kinase (Diagram 27.3). The inhibitor inactivates protein phosphatase-1 but has no effect on protein phosphatase-2A. In resting muscle, i.e. when glycogenolysis is not active, protein phosphatase inhibitor-1 is inactivated when it is dephosphorylated by protein phosphatase-2A (see Chart 28).

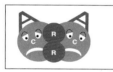

Diagram 27.1. Inactive cyclic AMP-dependent protein kinase.

Diagram 27.2. Very active phosphorylase kinase.

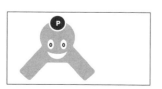

Diagram 27.3. Active protein phosphatase inhibitor-1.

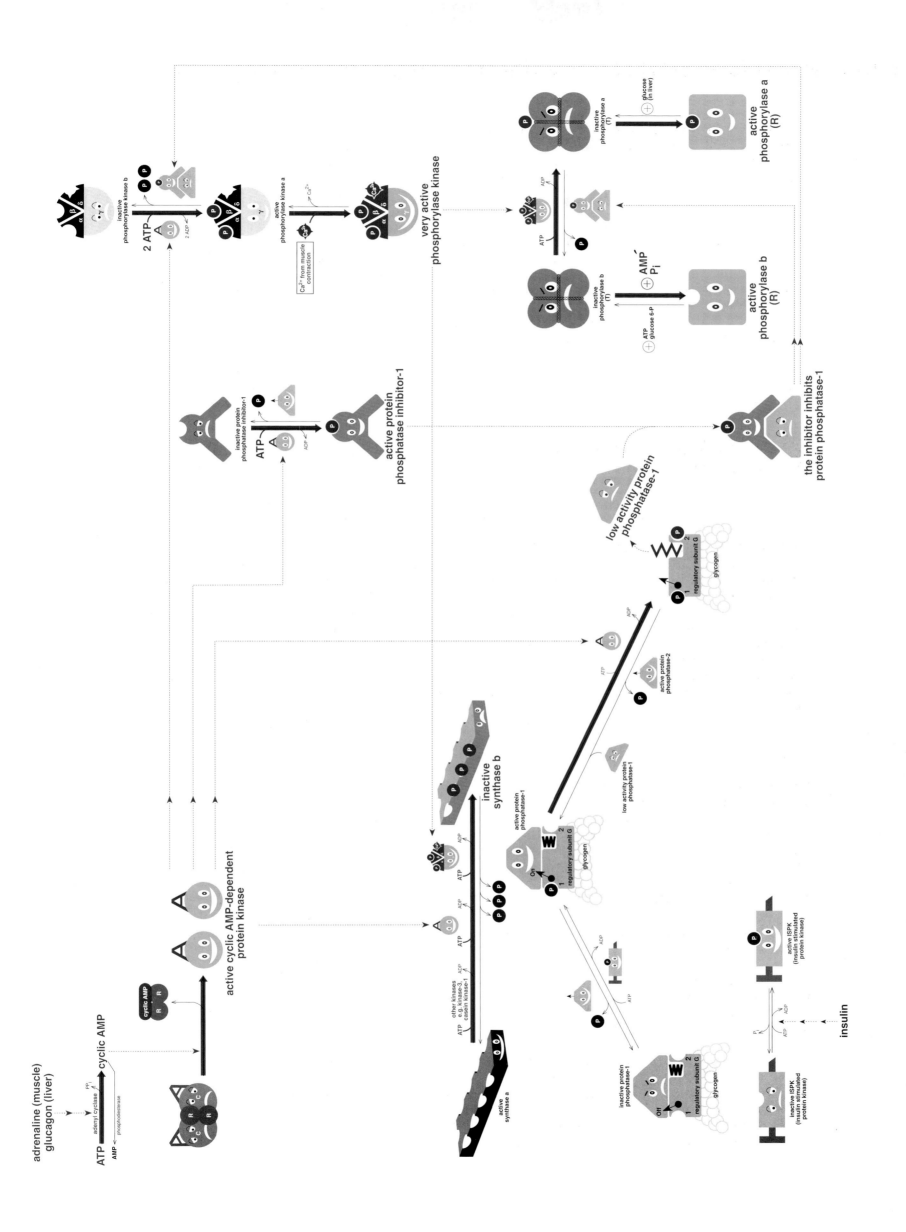

Glycogen metabolism, part IV: regulation of glycogen synthesis

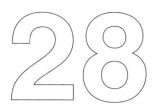

28

Chart 28 opposite. Regulation of glycogenesis.

Hormonal control: the role of insulin in the regulation of glycogen synthesis

Insulin is secreted by the β-cells of the pancreas following a carbohydrate meal. Insulin is needed to transport glucose into muscle cells, which means that glycogenesis is most active in the well-fed absorptive state. Having stressed the importance of insulin in regulating glycogen synthesis, it is something of an anticlimax to confess that many details of insulin action are imperfectly understood, in spite of much recent progress. However, fundamental to glycogen synthesis is the regulation of **glycogen synthase**, which is controlled as shown in Chart 28.

*Glycogen synthesis has been studied most extensively in muscle, and it is to this tissue that the following description of regulation relates. It should be noted that, whereas in the catabolic state of glycogenolysis phosphorylation by protein kinases dominates the scene, in the anabolic state of glycogenesis, the **protein phosphatases -1 and -2A** dominate and protein dephosphorylation occurs.*

Protein phosphatases

Protein phosphatase-1 and protein phosphatase-2A are the protein phosphatases in skeletal muscle that are involved in the regulation of glycogen metabolism.

Protein phosphatase-1 (PP-1)

Experiments suggest that this is a 37 kDa protein. It is inhibited by inhibitor-1 and by okadaic acid. There are several forms of PP-1, but the major active form which is associated with glycogen is known as PP-1G. This is a complex of PP-1 and a large, 160 kDa regulatory subunit G which is bound to glycogen.

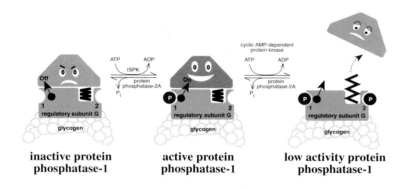

| inactive protein phosphatase-1 | active protein phosphatase-1 | low activity protein phosphatase-1 |

Regulation of PP-1G activity

PP-1G is active when phosphorylated at site 1 by insulin-stimulated protein kinase (ISPK). Conversely, it is slowly inactivated by dephosphorylation of site 1 by protein phosphatase-2A. However, PP-1 is also inactivated by phosphorylation at site 2 by cyclic AMP-dependent protein kinase, which causes the catalytic subunit to dissociate from the regulatory subunit G. The latter process is reversed by protein phosphatase-2A, which dephosphorylates site 2 permitting reassociation of the subunits to form active PP-1G.

Protein phosphatase-2A (PP-2A)

Several forms of PP-2A have been identified in eukaryotic cells, some containing two subunits and some three subunits. It is inhibited by okadaic acid but is not inhibited by inhibitor-1 (Diagram 28.1).

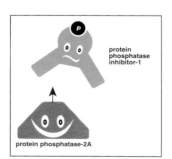

Diagram 28.1. Protein phosphatase-2A is not inhibited by protein phosphatase inhibitor-1.

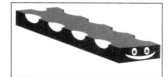

Diagram 28.2. Active glycogen synthase.

Chart 28: Regulation of glycogen synthesis
Removal of cyclic AMP

We have seen in the previous chapter how hormone-stimulated mobilization of glycogen is mediated by cyclic AMP. Obviously, if glycogen synthesis is to occur glycogen breakdown must stop, and so cyclic AMP must be destroyed. There is evidence based on studies of adipose tissue suggesting the presence of an insulin-stimulated series of reactions which results in the activation of **cyclic AMP phosphodiesterase** and conversion of cyclic AMP to AMP.

Insulin-stimulated protein kinase (ISPK)

Cohen's team in Dundee have described an insulin-stimulated protein kinase which activates **protein phosphatase-1 (PP-1)** in muscle. ISPK is thought to phosphorylate the glycogen-bound **regulatory subunit (G)** at site 1, thereby activating protein phosphatase-1.

Role of protein phosphatase-1 and 2A in regulating glycogenesis

With PP-1 active, glycogen synthesis can begin in earnest. Basically, PP-1 and PP-2A oppose the action of the protein kinases and they have the following effects:

1 Inactivation of PP-1. In resting muscle, PP-2A inactivates **PP-1** in an act of biochemical camaraderie which is much appreciated by its team mate, PP-1.

2 Inactivation of phosphorylase kinase. PP-1 dephosphorylates the β subunit, and PP-2A dephosphorylates the α subunit, thereby inactivating phosphorylase kinase. This prevents the formation of **phosphorylase a** thus inhibiting glycogen breakdown.

3 Activation of glycogen synthase. Finally, PP-1 dephosphorylates **synthase b** to form the high-activity **synthase a**, which catalyses the formation of glycogen from uridine diphosphate glucose.

Properties of glycogen synthase

Glycogen synthase is a simple tetramer of four identical 85 kDa subunits (for simplicity, a monomer is shown in Diagram 28.2). Its activity is regulated by synergistic phosphorylation, which can occur at nine sites (serine residues) in a precise, hierarchical manner producing the inactive **glycogen synthase b**. Glycogen synthase is most active in its dephosphorylated form, known as **synthase a**.

Inactivation (phosphorylation) of glycogen synthase

Glycogen synthase has 737 amino acid residues and, of these, nine are serine residues that can be phosphorylated. Two of these are situated in the N-terminal region of the molecule (N-7 and N-10) and seven are located in the C-terminal region (C-30, C-34, C-38, C-42, C-46, C-87 and C-100). It has been demonstrated *in vitro* that at least seven protein kinases can phosphorylate glycogen synthase; four important examples are:

1 Cyclic AMP-dependent protein kinase, which phosphorylates sites C-87, C-100 and N-7.

2 Glycogen synthase kinase-3, which phosphorylates the cluster of serine residues at C-30, C-34, C-38 and C-42 (but not C-46).

3 Phosphorylase kinase, which phosphorylates the serine residue at N-7.

4 Casein kinase-1, which phosphorylates at N-10.

5 Casein kinase-2, which phosphorylates at C-46.

Activation (dephosphorylation) of glycogen synthase by protein phosphatase-1

Protein phosphatase-1 dephosphorylates synthase b to produce active glycogen synthase a. Protein phosphatase-1 in turn requires activation by insulin-stimulated protein kinase (ISPK), as described above. ISPK causes **phosphorylation** of site 1 of the glycogen-bound regulatory subunit G, thereby activating protein phosphatase-1. Alternatively, **dephosphorylation** of site 2 of the regulatory subunit by protein phosphatase-2A allows reassociation of the catalytic and regulatory subunit to form active protein phosphatase-1.

Role of glucose in the inhibition of phosphorylase in liver

In liver, when glucose is abundant, it is the major inhibitor of phosphorylase activity. When glucose is bound to phosphorylase a, the latter acts as a better substrate for PP-1.

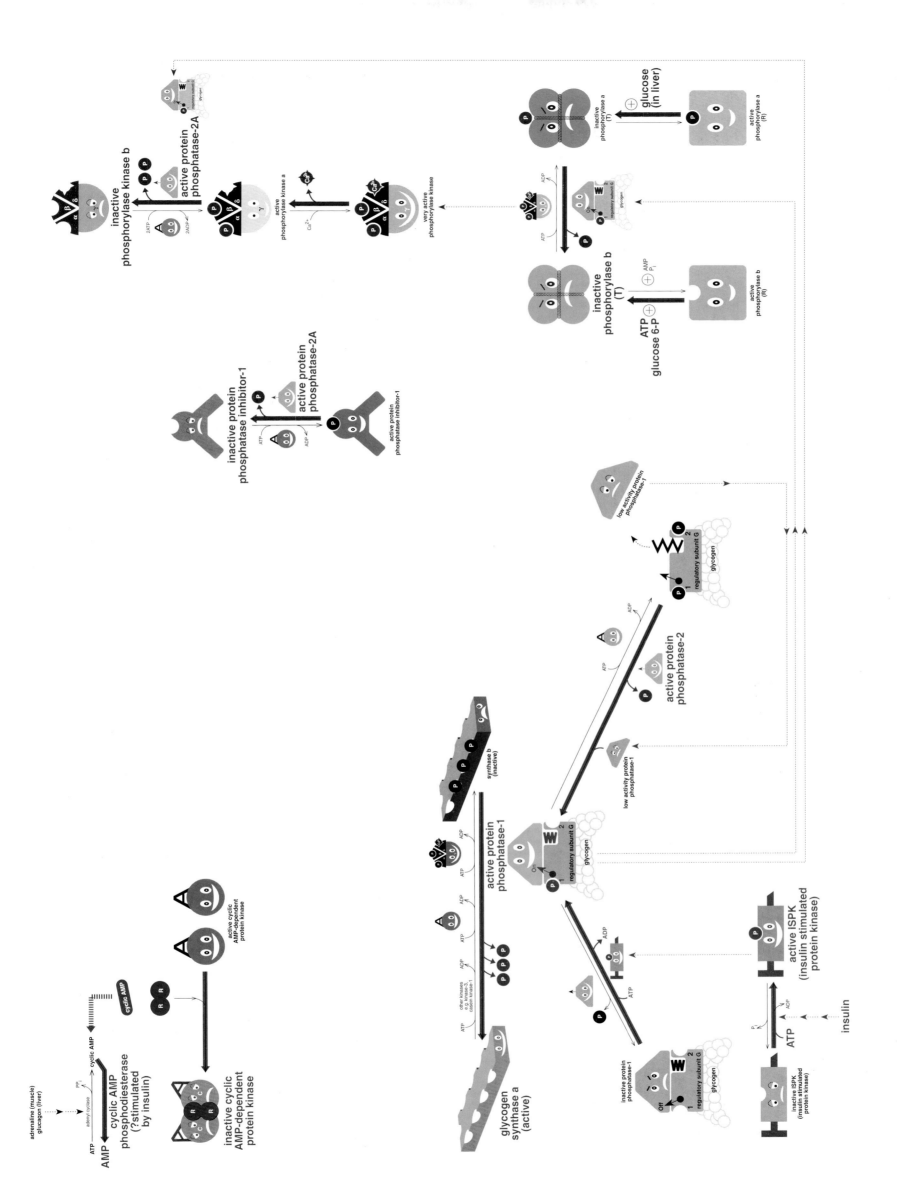

Regulation of glycolysis

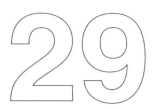

29

Chart 29 opposite. Regulation of glycolysis in muscle.

The regulatory mechanisms for glycolysis in liver and muscle are different

The glycolytic pathway is ubiquitous but its physiological significance can vary between different cell types. For example, there are marked differences between muscle and liver. Whereas glycolysis can be very important for energy metabolism in muscle (particularly anaerobically), glucose is not a major source of energy for the liver. On the contrary, liver in the well-fed state tends to convert glucose to the fuel reserves glycogen and triacylglycerols. Indeed, apart from during the phase of food absorption in the fed state, the liver is usually not in glycolytic mode, but instead **produces** glucose by either glycogenolysis or gluconeogenesis.

Chart 29: The regulatory stages in glycolysis
Transport of glucose into the cell

Glucose in the surrounding fluid must cross the plasma membrane into the cell. This occurs by facilitative diffusion mediated by a family of five proteins known as **facilitative glucose transporters**, which are distributed in different types of cells. Muscle cells and adipocytes, which are sensitive to insulin, have a transporter of the type known as Glu T4. In response to insulin these are recruited from vesicles within the cell to the plasma membrane, where they facilitate glucose uptake (see Chapter 5). It should be noted that the transporter in liver, Glu T2, does not need insulin to be active.

Phosphorylation of glucose

Phosphorylation of glucose to glucose 6-phosphate in the liver is catalysed by the glucose-phosphorylating isoenzyme, **glucokinase**, whereas in muscle the isoenzyme is **hexokinase**. Glucokinase (also known as hexokinase 4) is found only in liver and the pancreas, whereas hexokinase is widely distributed. The major difference between the isoenzymes is in their affinity for glucose. For glucokinase, the K_m (glucose) is 10 mmol/l, whereas for hexokinase it is 0.1 mmol/l. Thus the liver isoenzyme glucokinase is well adapted to cope with the high concentration surges of glucose in the blood during feeding. It should be remembered that dietary glucose from the intestines is absorbed into the hepatic portal vein, which transports the glucose directly to the liver at concentrations which can be greater than 20 mmol/l. On the other hand, the high affinity of hexokinase for glucose ensures that, even if the intracellular concentration of glucose in skeletal muscle should fall to as low as 0.1 mmol/l during a burst of strenuous exercise, the hexokinase reaction can still proceed at half its maximum velocity.

Another difference between hexokinase and glucokinase is that the former is inhibited by its product, glucose 6-phosphate, but not glucokinase. This ensures that, when the liver is presented with a large load of glucose, it can be phosphorylated to glucose 6-phosphate prior to glycogenesis or lipogenesis. On the other hand, if glucose 6-phosphate accumulates in muscle, it inhibits hexokinase, decreases the glycolytic flux and thereby conserves glucose.

Phosphofructokinase-1

For clarification purposes, this is known as phosphofructokinase-1 (PFK-1) to distinguish it from **phosphofructokinase-2 (PFK-2)**, which produces **fructose 2,6-bisphosphate (F 2,6-P_2)**. The latter is a potent allosteric stimulator of PFK-1.

ATP, although a substrate for PFK-1, is also an allosteric inhibitor when present in increased concentrations. This inhibition by ATP is potentiated by citrate. However, raised concentrations of its substrate, fructose 6-phosphate, can overcome this inhibition, thereby stimulating glycolysis.

Pyruvate kinase

The inhibitory effects of alanine and glucagon (mediated via cyclic AMP) on pyruvate kinase in liver are mainly concerned with directing the glycolytic pathway to the gluconeogenic mode. (**NB:** In muscle, alanine does not inhibit pyruvate kinase, and so pyruvate synthesis, and thus alanine, can be formed when the glucose alanine cycle is operating; see Chapter 18).

Fructose 1,6-bisphosphate activates pyruvate kinase allosterically by feedforward stimulation. This has obvious advantages for energy metabolism in exercising skeletal muscle by enhancing the glycolytic flux at the end of the pathway. In liver, this feedforward stimulatory effect of fructose 1,6-bisphosphate can overcome the inhibitory effect of alanine on pyruvate kinase.

Fructose 2,6-bisphosphate (F 2,6-P_2) is an important allosteric stimulator of glycolysis in muscle and inhibitor of gluconeogenesis in liver

Since F 2,6-P_2 stimulates PFK-1, it has an important influence on the rate of glycolysis. Furthermore, **in liver**, it inhibits fructose 1,6-bisphosphatase, thereby decreasing gluconeogenesis. The concentration of F 2,6-P_2 **in liver** is regulated by glucagon and **in muscle** by adrenaline. These hormones stimulate the production of cyclic AMP, which frees the active catalytic monomers of **cyclic AMP-dependent protein kinase** (see Chapter 27), which in turn phosphorylates the 'bifunctional enzyme' phosphofructokinase-2/fructose 2,6-bisphosphatase (PFK-2/FBPase-2). Following phosphorylation, **in muscle, PFK-2 is active** and FBPase-2 is inactive. This causes an increase in the concentration of F 2,6-P_2, which stimulates PFK-1, which increases the rate of glycolysis.

*NB: **In liver**, phosphorylation of the bifunctional enzyme has opposite effects: it **inactivates PFK-2** and **activates FBPase-2**. Thus in summary, **in liver**, glucagon causes concentrations of F 2,6-P_2 to be decreased; thus **PFK-1** activity is **decreased**, the inhibition of FBPase is relieved, and so gluconeogenesis is stimulated.*

The 'Pasteur effect'

Glucose can be metabolized *anaerobically* to generate ATP. This process demands a rapid flux of intermediates through the glycolytic pathway, but is a very inefficient route for generating ATP. In 1861, Louis Pasteur observed that when a normal oxygen supply was restored to yeast cells which had previously been respiring anaerobically, their demand for glucose was dramatically decreased. This inhibition of glycolysis by oxygen is known as the 'Pasteur effect'. It is due to a reduced flow of metabolites through glycolysis coupled to the more efficient oxidation of glucose by the Krebs cycle. It has since been observed in several tissues, including muscle, brain and liver. Metabolic crossover analysis indicates that regulation is at the phosphofructokinase-1 stage.

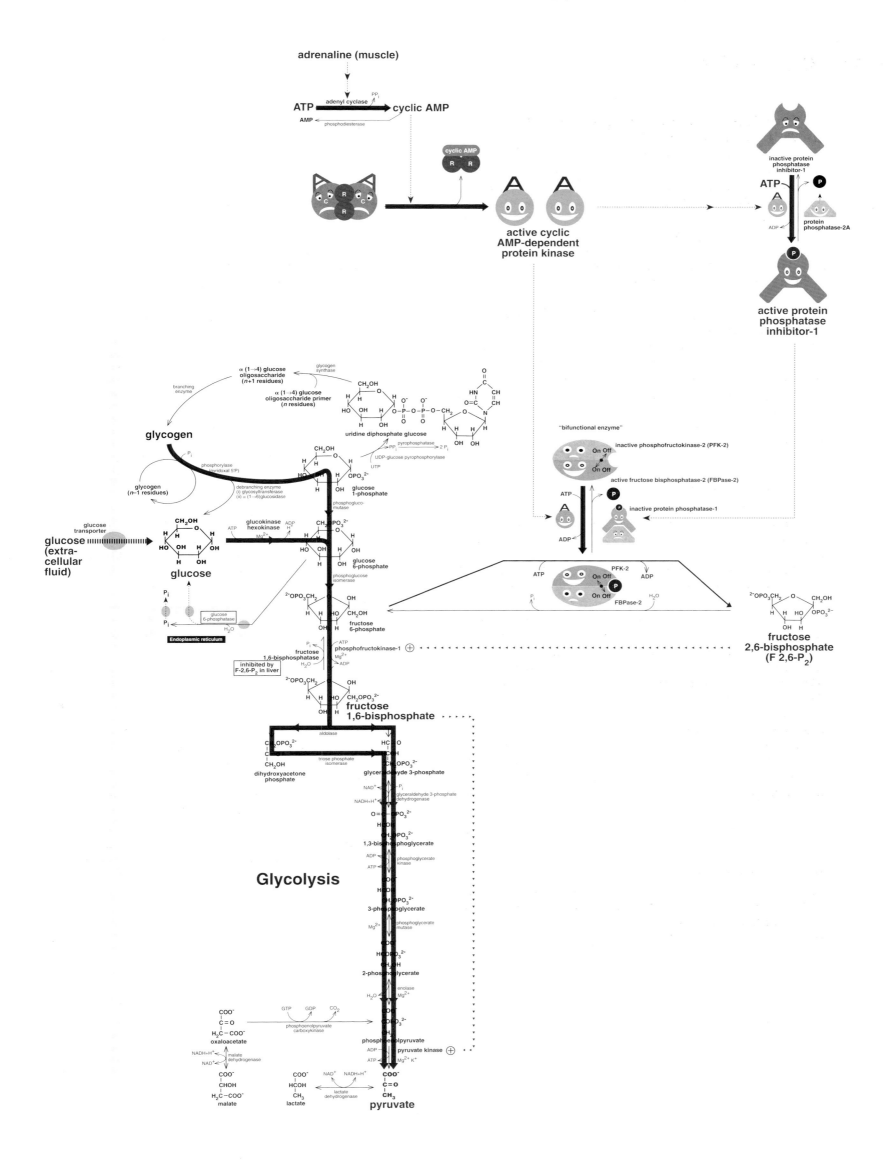

Regulation of the Krebs cycle

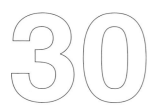

Chart 30 opposite. Regulation of Krebs cycle.

The Krebs cycle — the central junction of metabolism

The Krebs cycle is found in all mammalian cells, with the notable exception of mature red blood cells, which lack mitochondria. The cycle oxidizes acetyl CoA derived from carbohydrates, ketone bodies, fatty acids and amino acids, to produce $NADH+H^+$ and $FADH_2$ for ATP synthesis in the respiratory chain. Furthermore, components of the cycle form essential links with the pathways for gluconeogenesis, lipogenesis and amino acid metabolism. As such, regulation of the Krebs cycle must satisfy the diverse metabolic demands of these pathways in the various tissues with their different functions. For example, glucose is a premium fuel because of its vital role as a respiratory substrate for the brain and red blood cells. Because the body has a limited capacity to store carbohydrate, it must be conserved and not exhausted in a frenzied fit of exercise by the fuel-guzzling muscles which can very happily use fatty acids as an alternative energy source. PDH (pyruvate dehydrogenase) can therefore be thought of as the 'Minister for Glucose Conservation' since it determines whether or not pyruvate (which is mainly derived from carbohydrate or amino acids), enters the Krebs cycle for oxidation.

The activity of the Krebs cycle is controlled by the regulation of pyruvate dehydrogenase and isocitrate dehydrogenase.

Regulation of the pyruvate dehydrogenase (PDH) complex

Pyruvate dehydrogenase, although not a component of the Krebs cycle, has a commanding role in regulating the flux of glycolytic metabolites into the cycle. It is a multienzyme complex consisting of three component enzymes. These enzymes (E_1, pyruvate dehydrogenase, E_2, acetyl transferase, and E_3, dihydrolipoyl dehydrogenase) are responsible for decarboxylating the pyruvate, transferring the acetyl residue to CoA to form acetyl CoA, and oxidatively regenerating the intermediary lipoate involved. Associated with the complex are two enzymes which have regulatory roles (Diagram 30.1). One, namely PDH kinase, is a protein kinase which is specific for PDH. Its role is to phosphorylate and thus inactivate the pyruvate dehydrogenase component of the complex. The other, PDH phosphatase, is a specific PDH phosphatase which overcomes this inhibition by removing the phosphate groups, thereby

activating PDH. PDH is also regulated by the availability of its coenzymes $NADH+H^+$ and CoA, i.e. its activity is decreased when high ratios of $NADH+H^+/NAD^+$ and acetyl CoA/CoA prevail.

Diagram 30.1: Regulation of PDH by phosphorylation and dephosphorylation

When the energy charge of the cell is high, i.e. the ratio of ATP to ADP is increased, PDH kinase is active. E_1 is therefore phosphorylated at three sites and its activity is inhibited. Conversely, PDH kinase is inhibited by pyruvate, and this leads to activation of PDH in the presence of its substrate.

In muscle, PDH phosphatase is activated during muscle contraction, when cytosolic and mitochondrial concentrations of calcium ions are increased. In adipose tissue, PDH phosphatase is activated by insulin. In both of these cases, dephosphorylation of PDH occurs and PDH activity is stimulated.

Isocitrate dehydrogenase (ICDH)

ICDH is inhibited by the high ratio of $NADH+H^+/NAD$ which prevails in the high-energy state. When ICDH is inhibited, flux through this section of Krebs cycle is inhibited.

The purine nucleotide cycle

When large quantities of acetyl CoA are available for oxidation by the Krebs cycle, the availability of oxaloacetate for the citrate synthase reaction may become a rate-limiting factor. It is known that the purine nucleotide cycle (see Chart 30) is very active in muscle during exercise. This cycle generates fumarate from aspartate in the presence of GTP in circumstances when the AMP concentration is increased (e.g. when the ATP concentration is decreased, as during muscle contraction). The purine nucleotide cycle thus provides an anaplerotic supply of dicarboxylic acids, in particular oxaloacetate, in an effort to match the abundant supply of acetyl CoA presented for oxidation by Krebs cycle.

As would be expected, patients with muscle AMP deaminase deficiency (myoadenylate deaminase deficiency), suffer cramps and myalgias, and fatigue easily after exercise. AMP deaminase activity in the other tissues of these patients is normal.

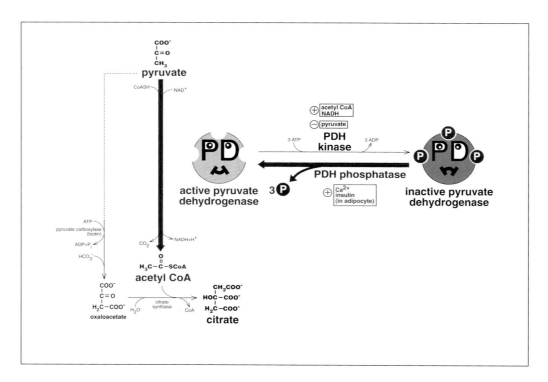

Diagram 30.1. Regulation of pyruvate dehydrogenase by phosphorylation and dephosphorylation.

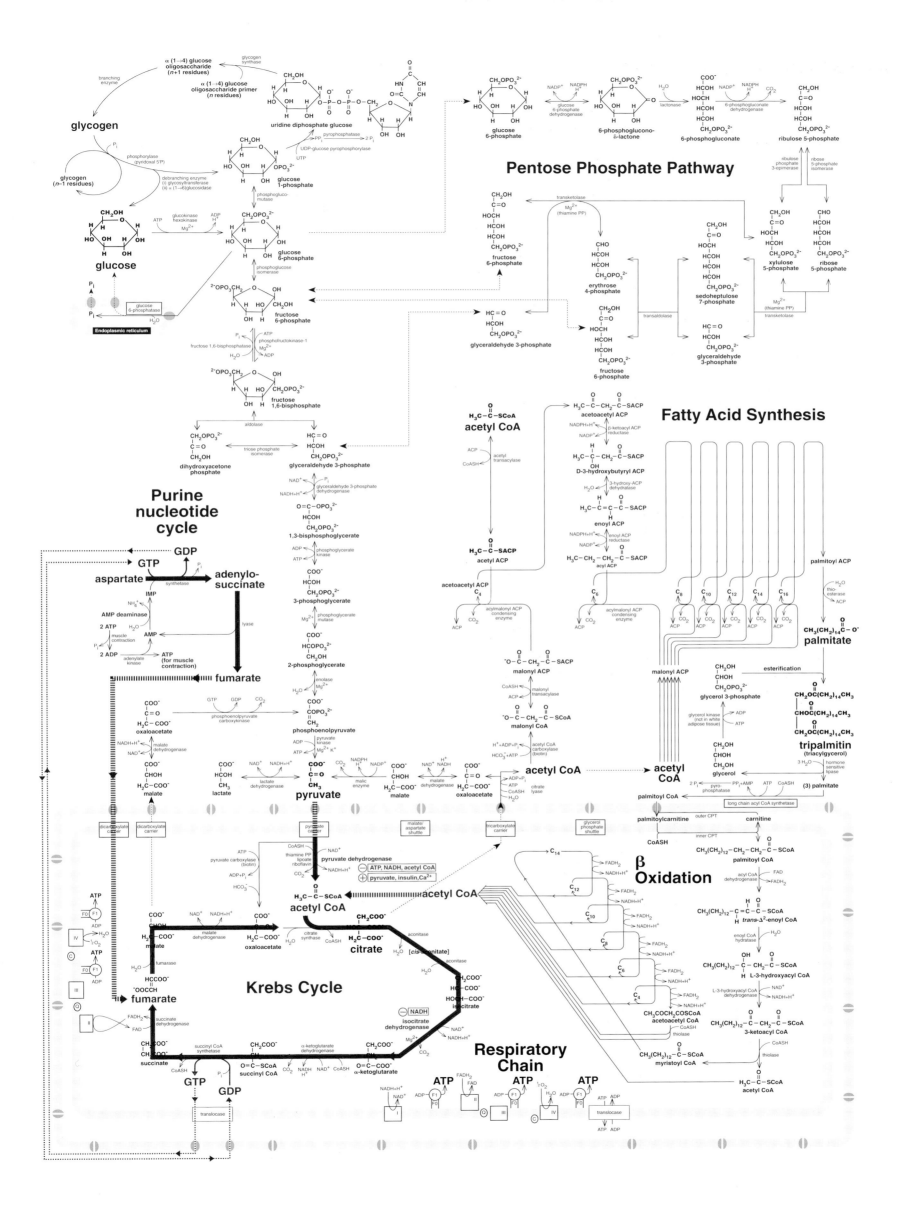

Regulation of gluconeogenesis

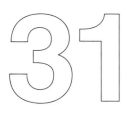

Chart 31 opposite. Regulation of gluconeogenesis.

Gluconeogenesis maintains the blood glucose concentration during fasting and starvation

The body's first and foremost reserve for maintaining the blood glucose concentration during fasting is liver glycogen. However, once this reserve is exhausted, glucose must be made from non-carbohydrate precursors. We have seen that the most abundant fuel reserve, the fatty acids in triacylglycerol, cannot be converted to glucose by mammals (see Chapter 14). However, glucose can be made from glycerol, lactate; and from amino acids formed by proteolysis of muscle proteins (see Chapters 8 and 18). This process is known as gluconeogenesis. It occurs mainly in the liver, but during prolonged starvation it is also active in kidney cortex.

Chart 31: Regulation of gluconeogenesis
Dependency of gluconeogenesis on the oxidation of fatty acids

Gluconeogenesis, which operates during starvation, is linked to the mobilization of fat and the oxidation of fatty acids. The latter results in the formation in the mitochondrion of large amounts of acetyl CoA, NADH+H$^+$ and ATP, with the following effects on mitochondrial reactions:

1 Isocitrate dehydrogenase is inhibited by NADH+H$^+$.

2 Pyruvate dehydrogenase is inhibited by acetyl CoA, ATP and NADH+H$^+$.

3 Pyruvate carboxylase is stimulated by acetyl CoA.

4 The equilibrium of the mitochondrial **malate dehydrogenase** reaction is displaced to favour the reduction of oxaloacetate to malate.

5 ATP (and GTP via the nucleoside diphosphate kinase reaction) from the β-oxidation and respiratory chain pathways is used as a cosubstrate for the pyruvate carboxylase, phosphoenolpyruvate carboxykinase and phosphoglycerate kinase reactions.

Gluconeogenic precursors

Amino acids, particularly **alanine**, are important gluconeogenic precursors, but they must first be metabolized to cytosolic oxaloacetate (see Chapter 20). **Glycerol**, derived from triacylglycerol, is also an important gluconeogenic precursor. It is phosphorylated in the liver by **glycerol kinase** to form glycerol 3-phosphate, which in turn is oxidized by glycerol 3-phosphate dehydrogenase to form the gluconeogenic intermediate **dihydroxyacetone phosphate**. Finally, **lactate**, produced for example by anaerobic glycolysis in red blood cells or muscle, is also used for gluconeogenesis.

Hormonal regulation of gluconeogenesis

Glucagon is an important hormone in the early fasting state. It stimulates **hormone-sensitive lipase** through the action of cyclic AMP-dependent protein kinase. Furthermore, it stimulates fructose 1,6-bisphosphatase and inhibits pyruvate kinase by the same mechanism. Glucagon also has effects on the synthesis of certain enzymes. It increases synthesis of the aminotransferases, phosphoenolpyruvate carboxykinase and glucose 6-phosphatase, which favour gluconeogenesis.

Regulatory enzymes
Pyruvate carboxylase

Pyruvate carboxylase, which converts pyruvate to oxaloacetate, is stimulated by acetyl CoA. (**NB:** Pyruvate dehydrogenase, which competes for pyruvate as a substrate, is **inactivated** by acetyl CoA.)

Phosphoenolpyruvate carboxykinase (PEPCK)

PEPCK decarboxylates oxaloacetate to phosphoenolpyruvate (PEP). It requires GTP, which can be obtained from ATP by the nucleoside diphosphate kinase reaction. PEPCK activity is induced in the long term when the ratio of glucagon to insulin is high.

In theory, PEP could be converted to pyruvate, enter the Krebs cycle as oxaloacetate and be reconverted to PEP in a futile cycle. This does not happen, because liver pyruvate kinase is inactivated by cyclic AMP-dependent protein kinase (due to the presence of glucagon), and is inhibited by alanine which is present in increased concentrations during gluconeogenic conditions (see Chapter 18).

Fructose 1,6-bisphosphatase (F1,6-BPase)

Regulation of this enzyme has been mentioned in Chapter 29. F1,6-BPase is inhibited by fructose 2,6-bisphosphate (F2,6-P$_2$). Glucagon, which is secreted by the α cells of the pancreas in response to a low blood glucose concentration, stimulates the breakdown of F2,6-P$_2$ through the action of cAMP-dependent protein kinase. Removal of the allosteric inhibitor F2,6-P$_2$ results in F1,6-BPase activity being stimulated.

Glucose 6-phosphatase

Glucose 6-phosphatase is located on the luminal surface of the endoplasmic reticulum in liver cells (see Diagram 31.1). Its substrate, glucose 6-phosphate, is transported from the cytosol by a translocator into the lumen of the endoplasmic reticulum, where it is hydrolysed to glucose and P$_i$. The reaction products are then transported into the cytosol by a glucose translocator and a P$_i$ translocator.

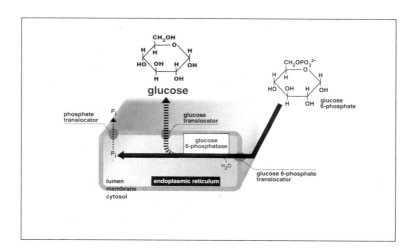

Diagram 31.1. Glucose 6-phosphatase is localized on the inside of the rough endoplasmic reticulum membrane. **NB:** The ribosomes are not shown.

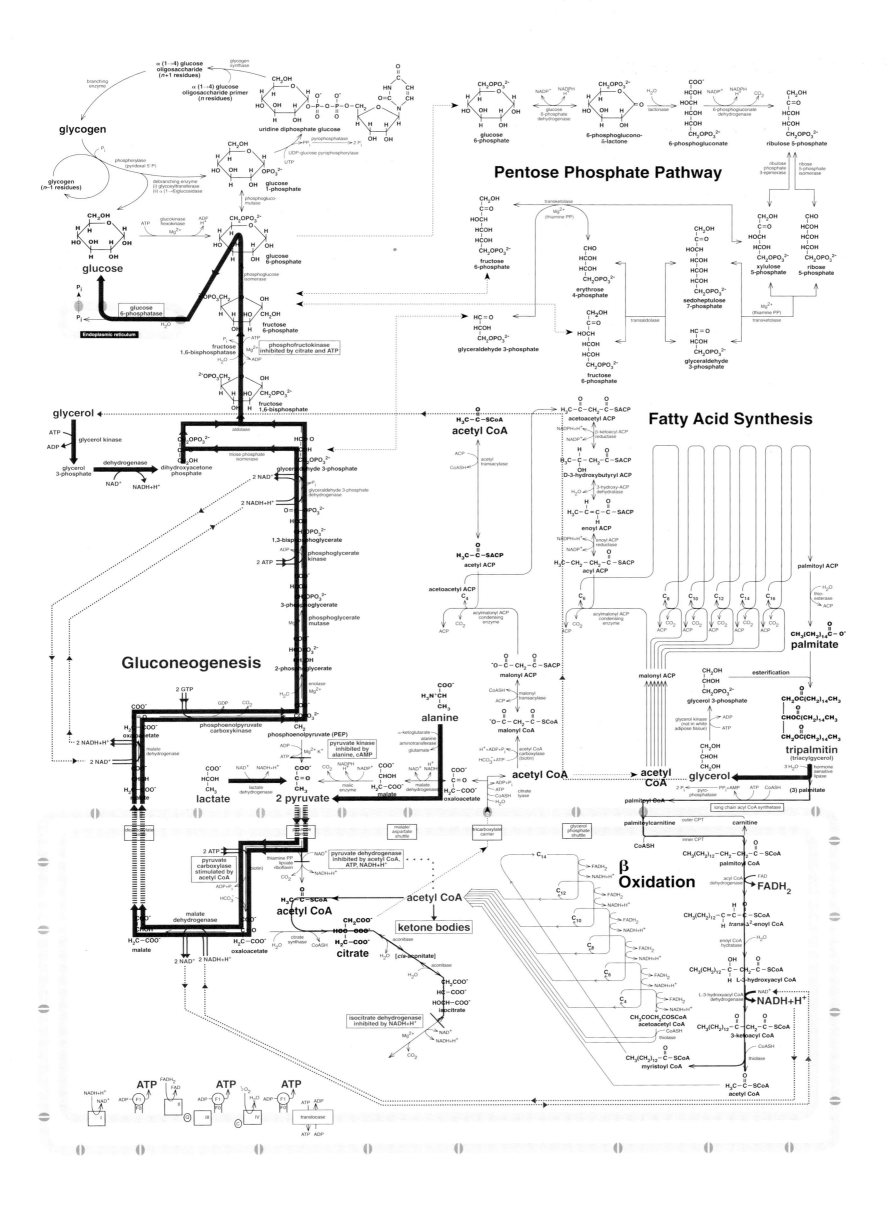

Regulation of fatty acid oxidation, part I: mobilization of fatty acids from storage in adipose tissue

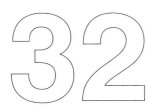

Diagram 32.1 opposite. The triacylglycerol/fatty acid cycle.

Diagram 32.2. Mobilization of fatty acids in adipose tissue.

During exercise, periods of stress or starvation, the triacylglycerol reserves in adipose tissue are mobilized as fatty acids for oxidation as a respiratory fuel. This is analogous to the mobilization of glycogen as glucose units; it occurs under similar circumstances, and is under similar hormonal control.

Fatty acids are a very important energy substrate in red muscle, and also in liver, where they are metabolized to the ketone bodies. Because fatty acids are hydrophobic, they are transported in the blood bound to albumin. They can serve most cells as a respiratory fuel, with the notable exceptions of brain and red blood cells, which lack the enzymes for fatty acid oxidation.

Regulation of the utilization of fatty acids appears to be at four levels:

1 Lipolysis of triacylglycerol to form the free fatty acids;

2 Re-esterification of the fatty acids, or alternatively their mobilization from adipose tissue;

3 Transport of the acyl CoA esters into the mitochondrion;

4 Availability of FAD and NAD$^+$+H$^+$ for β-oxidation.

The first two of these will be considered now and the other two will be covered in Chapter 33.

Lipolysis in adipose tissue

Lipolysis in adipose tissue is controlled by **hormone-sensitive lipase**. Other synonyms for this enzyme are 'triacylglycerol lipase' and 'mobilizing lipase'. This enzyme hydrolyses triacylglycerol to monoacylglycerol which in turn is hydrolysed by **monoacylglycerol lipase**. In Diagram 32.1, for example, **tripalmitin** is converted to **three molecules of palmitate** and **glycerol**.

Lipolysis is stimulated by adrenaline during exercise, by glucagon during fasting, and by adrenocorticotropin (ACTH) during starvation (Diagram 32.2). The mechanism involves cyclic AMP-dependent protein kinase, as described in Chapter 27, which both stimulates hormone-sensitive lipase and inhibits acetyl CoA carboxylase. Furthermore, as a long-term adaptation to prolonged starvation, cortisol stimulates the synthesis of hormone-sensitive lipase, thereby increasing its concentration and activity. Conversely, in the well-fed state, hormone-sensitive lipase is inhibited by insulin.

Mobilization of fatty acids: the triacylglycerol–fatty acid cycle

We have seen how triacylglycerol is hydrolysed by hormone-sensitive lipase to **free fatty acids** and **glycerol**. However, glycerol kinase is absent from white adipose tissue and so the glycerol cannot be metabolized further. Instead, it goes to the liver where hepatic glycerol kinase forms glycerol 3-phosphate, which undergoes gluconeogenesis.

In adipose tissue, the **free fatty acids** liberated by lipolysis have two possible fates within the adipocyte:

1 They can be released from the adipocyte for β-oxidation elsewhere, e.g. by muscle or liver.

2 Alternatively, the fatty acids can be re-esterified with **glycerol 3-phosphate**. This is illustrated in Diagram 32.1, which shows how fatty acids (e.g. palmitate) are activated by acyl CoA synthetase to form acyl CoA. This then combines first with glycerol 3-phosphate to form lysophosphatidate, then proceeds via other intermediates, as shown in the diagram, to form triacylglycerol.

The importance of insulin in maintaining this cycle should be noted. The Glu T4 glucose transporter in adipose tissue needs insulin to be effective, therefore during fasting the cycle is disrupted. As a result, glycerol 3-phosphate is not formed by glycolysis and so is not available for re-esterification of the fatty acids formed by hormone-sensitive lipase. Consequently, in the absence of insulin, these free fatty acids are released from the adipocyte for use as a respiratory fuel by the tissues.

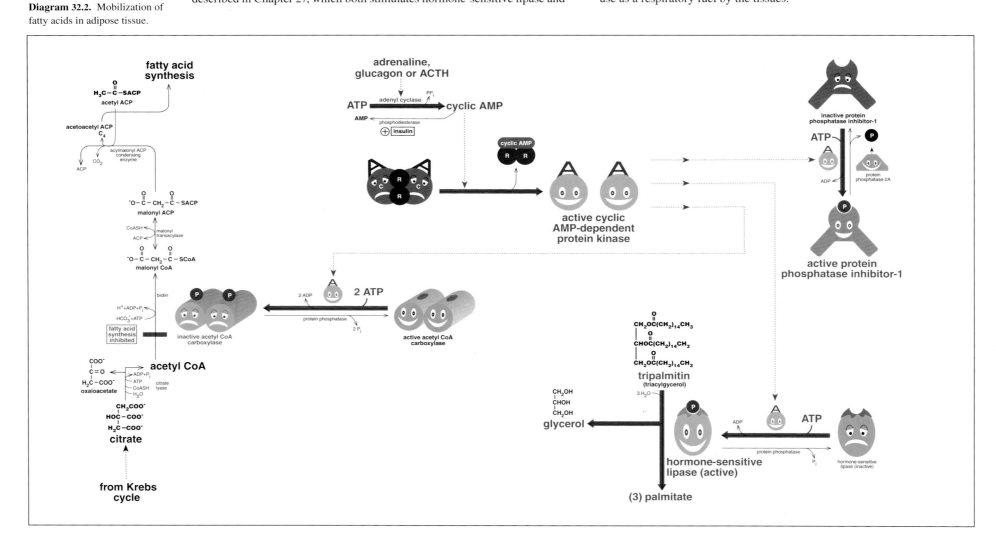

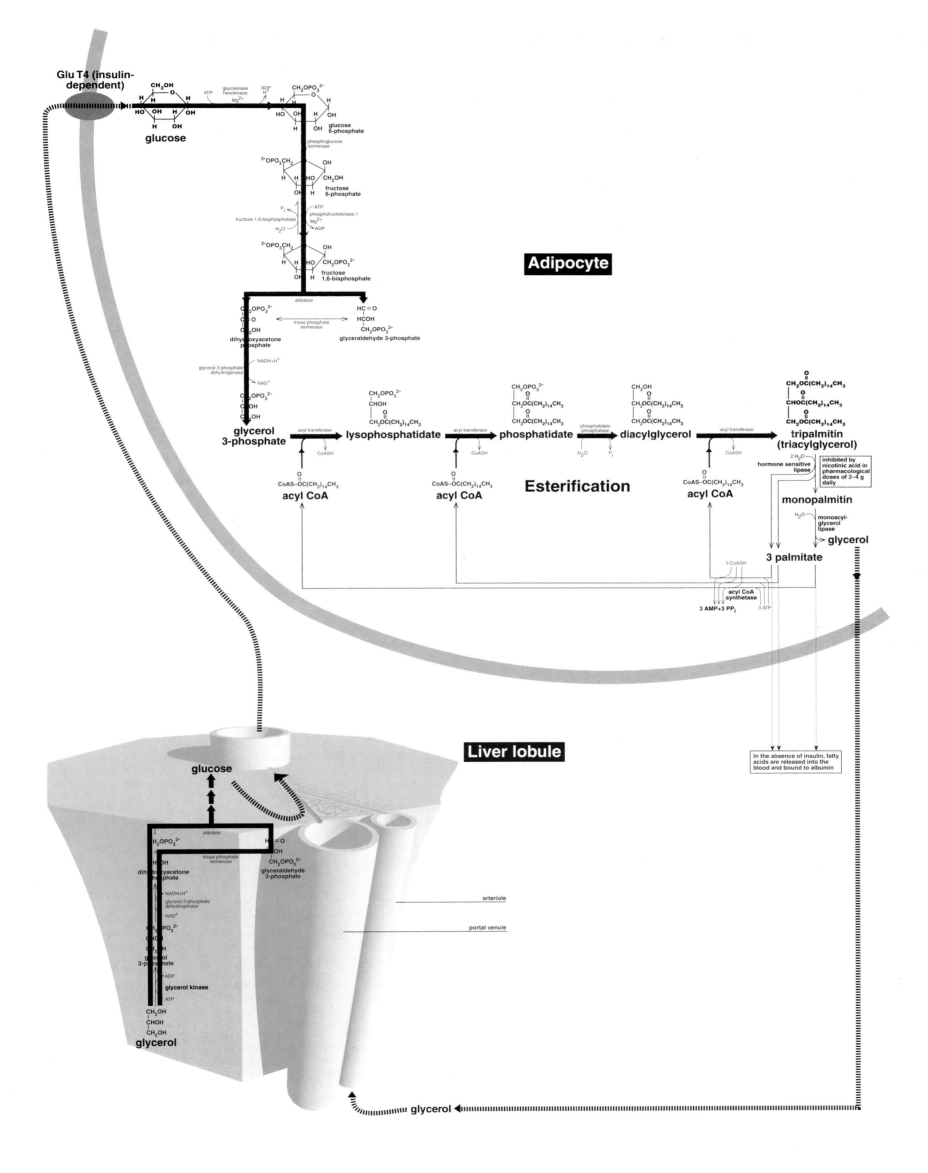

Glu T4 (insulin-dependent)

glucose

Adipocyte

glucokinase
hexokinase
Mg²⁺

ATP

ADP
H⁺

glucose
6-phosphate

phosphoglucose
isomerase

fructose
6-phosphate

fructose 1,6-bisphosphatase

ATP
phosphofructokinase-1
Mg²⁺
ADP

Pᵢ
H₂O

fructose
1,6-bisphosphate

aldolase

dihydroxyacetone
phosphate

triose phosphate
isomerase

glyceraldehyde 3-phosphate

glycerol 3-phosphate
dehydrogenase

NADH+H⁺

NAD⁺

**glycerol
3-phosphate**

acyl transferase

CoASH

lysophosphatidate

acyl transferase

CoASH

phosphatidate

phosphatidate
phosphatase

H₂O

Pᵢ

diacylglycerol

acyl transferase

CoASH

**tripalmitin
(triacylglycerol)**

Esterification

CoAS–OC(CH₂)₁₄CH₃

acyl CoA

CoAS–OC(CH₂)₁₄CH₃

acyl CoA

CoAS–OC(CH₂)₁₄CH₃

acyl CoA

2 H₂O

hormone sensitive
lipase

inhibited by
nicotinic acid in
pharmacological
doses of 2–4 g
daily

monopalmitin

H₂O

monoacyl-
glycerol
lipase

glycerol

3 palmitate

3 CoASH

acyl CoA
synthetase

3 AMP+3 PPᵢ   3 ATP

In the absence of insulin, fatty
acids are released into the
blood and bound to albumin

Liver lobule

glucose

aldolase

dihydroxyacetone
phosphate

triose phosphate
isomerase

glyceraldehyde
3-phosphate

NADH+H⁺

glycerol 3-phosphate
dehydrogenase

NAD⁺

glycerol
3-phosphate

ADP

glycerol kinase

ATP

CH₂OH
CHOH
CH₂OH
glycerol

arteriole

portal venule

glycerol

Regulation of fatty acid oxidation, part II: the carnitine shuttle

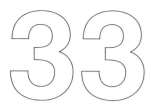

The release of fatty acids from triacylglycerols in adipose tissue is regulated by hormone-sensitive lipase (Chapter 32). The fatty acids, bound to albumin, are then transported to the liver and muscles for utilization. The rate of uptake by these tissues of the fatty acids is proportional to their concentration in the blood. Thereafter, the rate of β-oxidation is regulated by:
1 The carnitine shuttle for the mitochondrial uptake of fatty acids;
2 Availability of the coenzymes NAD$^+$ and FAD.

Chart 33 opposite. The carnitine shuttle and the β-oxidation of fatty acids.

Diagram 33.1. The carnitine shuttle.

Transport of activated fatty acids into the mitochondrial matrix by the carnitine shuttle is inhibited by malonyl CoA

Fatty acids are activated by long chain acyl CoA synthetase to form acyl CoA, e.g. **palmitoyl CoA** as shown in Chart 33 and Diagram 33.1. A transport system, the **carnitine shuttle**, is needed for long-chain fatty acids to cross the inner mitochondrial membrane. In liver, this transport is inhibited by **malonyl CoA**. Since malonyl CoA is produced during fatty acid synthesis, this ensures that the newly formed fatty acids are not immediately transported into the mitochondrion and broken down.

The carnitine carrier system consists of **carnitine/acyl-carnitine translocase** and two carnitine-palmitoyl-transferases (CPT): an **outer CPT I** and an **inner CPT II**.

Many textbooks show the inner and outer CPTs located on the inner and outer sides of the inner membrane. Diagram 33.1, based on evidence by Murthy and Pande (1987), suggests that, although the inner CPT resides on the inner side of the inner membrane, the outer CPT is located on the inner side of the **outer** membrane. This model is attractive because it enables easy interaction between the **malonyl-CoA binding site** and the outer CPT.

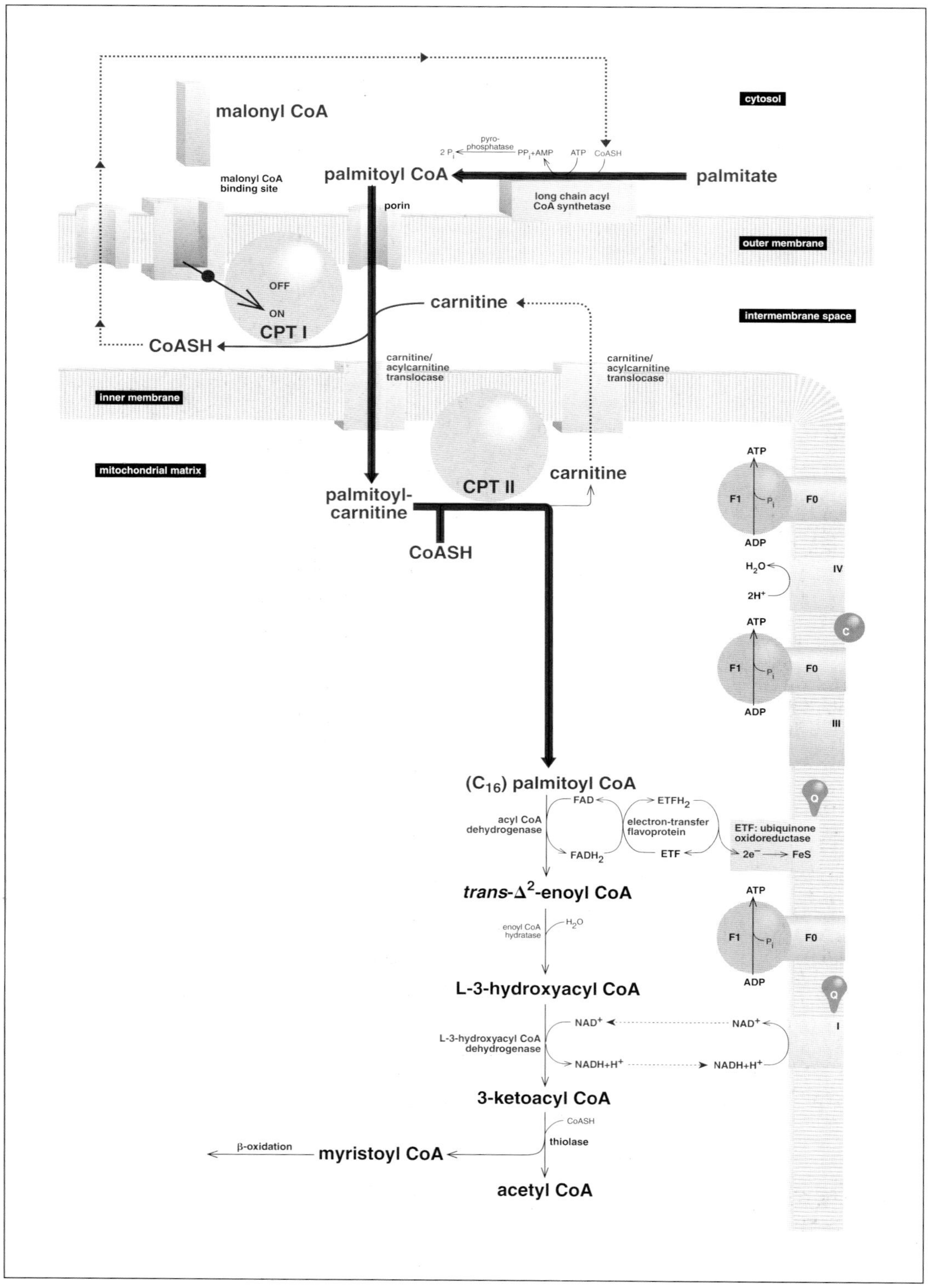

Availability of FAD and NAD$^+$ for β-oxidation

The L-3-hydroxyacyl-CoA dehydrogenase of β-oxidation requires NAD$^+$ as coenzyme. However, it has to compete with the three NAD$^+$-dependent dehydrogenases of the Krebs cycle for the limited NAD$^+$ available. In the high-energy state, when both pathways are highly active, β-oxidation may be limited by the supply of NAD$^+$. This may be an important rate-limiting factor especially in muscle.

Likewise, acyl CoA dehydrogenase needs a supply of FAD for activity which must be regenerated from FADH$_2$ by oxidation via the 'electron transfer flavoprotein' and the respiratory chain.

Acyl-CoA dehydrogenase and hypoglycaemia

Mitochondria contain three FAD-dependent, acyl CoA dehydrogenases which act on long-, medium- and short-chain fatty acids, although there is some overlap of specificities. In the process FAD is reduced to FADH$_2$ and the electrons are transferred to another FAD prosthetic group of the **electron-transfer flavoprotein (ETF)**, which is a soluble matrix protein (Diagram 33.1). The electrons now pass to **ETF: ubiquinone oxidoreductase** before passing to ubiquinone and entering the respiratory chain.

Medium-chain acyl CoA dehydrogenase deficiency
Sudden infant death syndrome

The sudden unexplained death of an infant is known as a 'cot death' or 'sudden infant death syndrome' (SIDS). In a few cases of SIDS, a possible cause is deficiency of medium-chain acyl CoA dehydrogenase. In this condition, β-oxidation is restricted and so there is increased oxidation of glucose as a respiratory fuel to meet the demands for energy. If the reserves of glycogen become exhausted, this may result in fatal hypoglycaemia.

Forbidden fruit—the unripe ackee and Jamaican vomiting sickness

In Jamaica, it is widely known that the unripe fruit of the ackee tree is to be avoided. Those who disregard the warning and eat the fruit experience an acute vomiting attack and suffer a syndrome known as Jamaican vomiting sickness. The ackee tree (*Blighia sapida* after Captain Bligh of 'Mutiny on the Bounty' fame) bears a fruit which, when ripe, is widely eaten in Jamaica. The unripe fruit, however, contains an unusual α-amino acid called hypoglycin A (methylenecyclopropylalanine, MCPA). Hypoglycin A is metabolized to methylenecyclopropylacetate, which undergoes activation by acyl CoA synthetase to form MCPA-CoA, which inhibits acyl CoA dehydrogenase. Consequently, β-oxidation is suppressed and glucose must be oxidized instead. Once the glycogen reserves are exhausted, hypoglycaemia rapidly follows. Before this hypoglycaemia was recognized, thousands of deaths were caused by ackee poisoning.

Reference

Murthy M.S.R. and Pande S.V., Malonyl CoA binding site and the overt carnitine palmitoyl transferase activity reside on opposite sides of the outer mitochondrial membrane. *Proc Natl Acad Sci USA* **84**, 378–382, 1987.

Chart / Diagram labels

malonyl CoA

cytosol

pyro-phosphatase

2 P$_i$ PP$_i$+AMP ATP CoASH

malonyl CoA binding site

palmitoyl CoA

palmitate

porin

long chain acyl CoA synthetase

outer membrane

OFF
ON
CPT I

carnitine

intermembrane space

CoASH

carnitine/acylcarnitine translocase

carnitine/acylcarnitine translocase

inner membrane

mitochondrial matrix

palmitoyl-carnitine

CPT II

carnitine

CoASH

ATP
F1 P$_i$ F0
ADP

H$_2$O
2H$^+$
IV

ATP
F1 P$_i$ F0
ADP

III

(C$_{16}$) palmitoyl CoA

FAD   ETFH$_2$

acyl CoA dehydrogenase

electron-transfer flavoprotein

ETF: ubiquinone oxidoreductase

FADH$_2$ ETF   2e$^-$ FeS

trans-Δ^2-enoyl CoA

enoyl CoA hydratase H$_2$O

ATP
F1 P$_i$ F0
ADP

L-3-hydroxyacyl CoA

NAD$^+$ NAD$^+$

L-3-hydroxyacyl CoA dehydrogenase

NADH+H$^+$ NADH+H$^+$

I

3-ketoacyl CoA

CoASH
thiolase

β-oxidation   myristoyl CoA

acetyl CoA

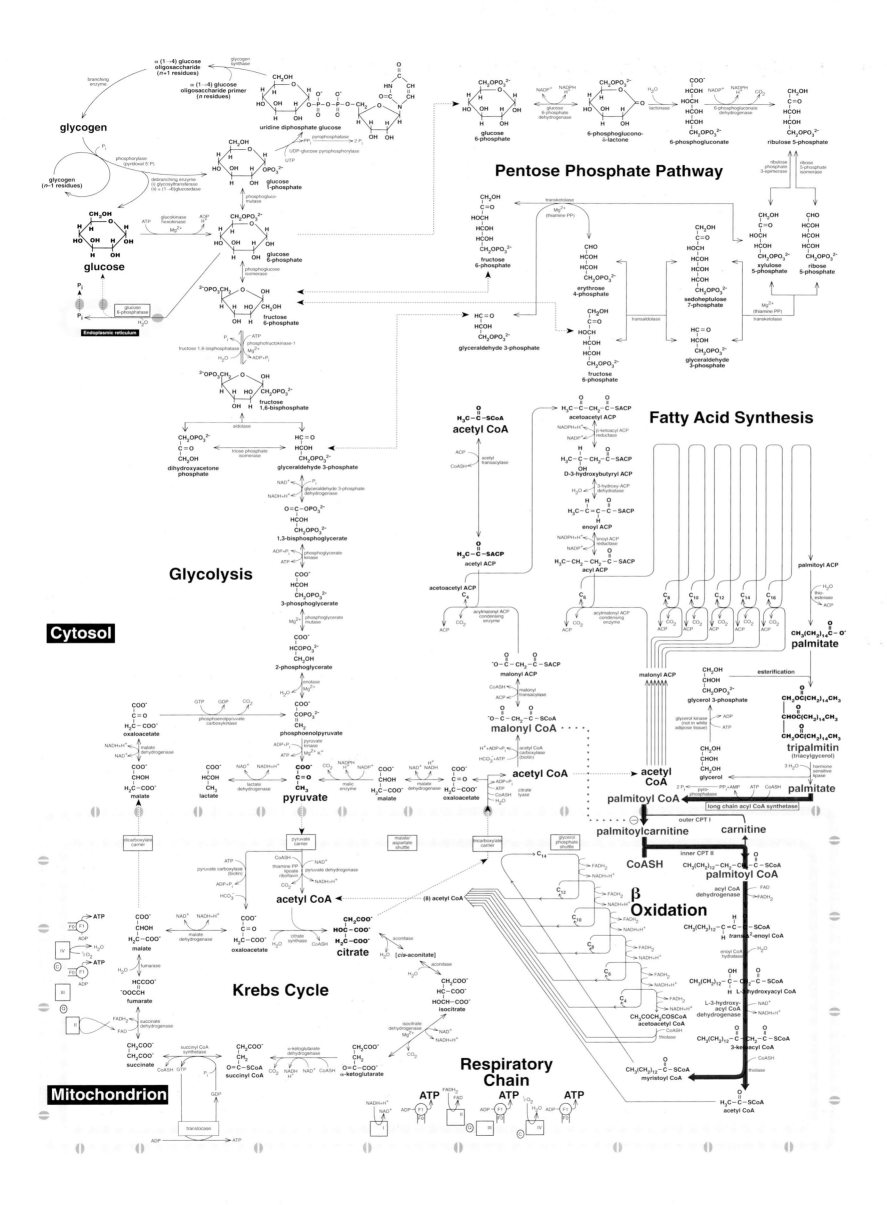

The ketone bodies

34

Chart 34 opposite. Ketogenesis.

The misunderstood 'villains' of metabolism

Diabetic patients know that the detection in their urine of the 'ketone bodies' (namely D-3-hydroxybutyrate, acetoacetate and acetone) is a danger signal that their diabetes is poorly controlled. Indeed, in severely uncontrolled diabetes, if the ketone bodies are produced in massive supranormal quantities they are associated with ketoacidosis. In this life-threatening complication of diabetes mellitus, the acids D-3-hydroxybutyric acid and acetoacetic acid are produced rapidly, causing high concentrations of protons which overwhelm the body's acid–base buffering system, with the consequential dangerous decrease in blood pH. It is this low pH due to the protons which is so harmful, and not the ketone bodies themselves.

Until the middle of the 1960s, it was thought that the ketone bodies were 'metabolic garbage' with no beneficial physiological role. However, it is now realized that, during starvation, the brain uses the ketone bodies as a fuel in addition to its usual fuel glucose. This **regulated and controlled** production of the ketone bodies causes a state known as '**ketosis**'. In ketosis the blood pH remains buffered within normal limits. This is a very important glucose-sparing (and therefore tissue-protein conserving) adaptation to starvation which compensates for exhaustion of the glycogen reserves. (It should be remembered that the brain cannot use fatty acids as a fuel.)

Chart 34: Ketogenesis

During starvation, prolonged severe exercise or uncontrolled diabetes, the rate of production of the ketone bodies is increased. The most important precursors for ketogenesis are fatty acids derived from triacylglycerol. However, certain amino acids (leucine, isoleucine, lysine, phenylalanine, tyrosine and tryptophan) are also ketogenic.

Ketogenesis from triacylglycerols

The ketone bodies are produced in liver mitochondria from **fatty acids** which in turn are produced by the action of **hormone-sensitive lipase** on **triacylglycerols** stored in adipose tissue. The fatty acids are subjected to β-oxidation to form **acetyl CoA**. The interdependent relationship between the pathways for β-oxidation and gluconeogenesis is emphasized in Chapter 31 and is illustrated in Chart 34, which shows how mitochondrial **oxaloacetate** is diverted towards gluconeogenesis. Hence, oxaloacetate, which is needed

Diagram 34.1. Fatty acid mobilization from adipose tissue for ketogenesis in the liver.

by the **citrate synthase** reaction for acetyl CoA to enter the Krebs cycle, is directed away from the mitochondrion to the cytosol for gluconeogenesis. Consequently, there is an increased flux of acetyl CoA through **acetoacetyl CoA thiolase** towards ketogenesis.

Ketogenesis involves the **acetoacetyl CoA thiolase** reaction, which combines two molecules of acetyl CoA to form **acetoacetyl CoA**. This in turn is condensed with a third acetyl CoA by **HMGCoA synthase** to form 3-hydroxy-3-methylglutaryl-CoA (**HMGCoA**) (see Chart 34). Finally, HMGCoA is cleaved by **lyase** to form **acetoacetate** and acetyl CoA. The NADH formed by the L-3-hydroxyacyl CoA dehydrogenase reaction of β-oxidation could be coupled to the reduction of acetoacetate to **D-3-hydroxybutyrate**, thereby regenerating NAD^+. Acetone is produced by non-enzymic decarboxylation of acetoacetate, and is formed in relatively small proportions compared with the acids.

The rate of ketogenesis is coupled to the supply of fatty acids and the regulation of β-oxidation, as described in Chapters 32 and 33.

The ketone bodies are thought to leave the mitochondrion, in exchange for pyruvate, by a carrier mechanism.

Ketogenesis from amino acids

Certain amino acids can wholly or partially be used for ketogenesis. The details of these pathways are shown in Chapters 18 and 19. Entry to ketogenesis is either at acetyl CoA (isoleucine), acetoacetate (phenylalanine and tyrosine), HMGCoA (leucine) or acetoacetyl CoA (lysine and tryptophan), as outlined in Chart 34.

Diagram 34.1: Fatty acids are mobilized from adipose tissue for ketogenesis in the liver

In the ketotic state, hormone-sensitive lipase is active and triacylglycerols are hydrolysed to glycerol and fatty acids. The liberated fatty acids leave the adipocyte and diffuse into the blood, where they are bound to albumin and transported to the liver. In the liver, β-oxidation and ketogenesis occur. The 'ketone bodies', acetoacetate and D-3-hydroxybutyrate produced are exported as fuel for tissue oxidation, especially by muscle and by the brain.

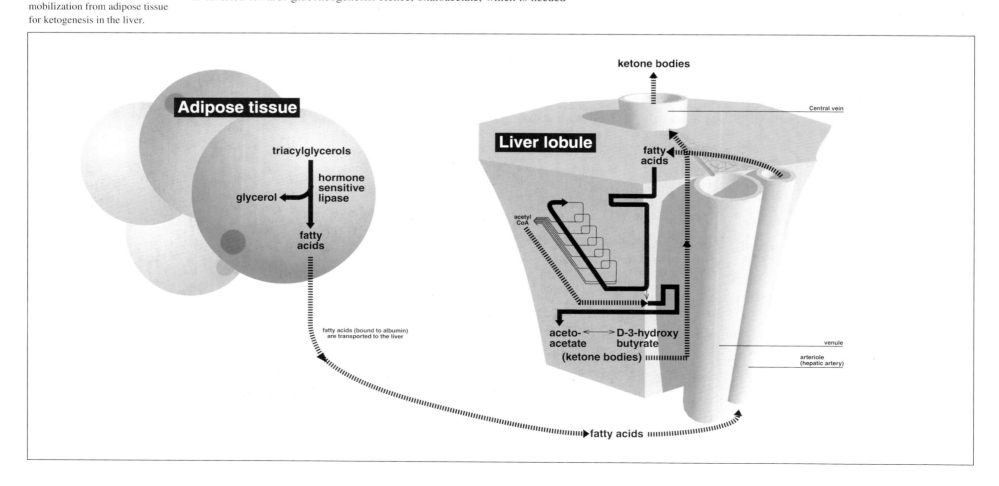

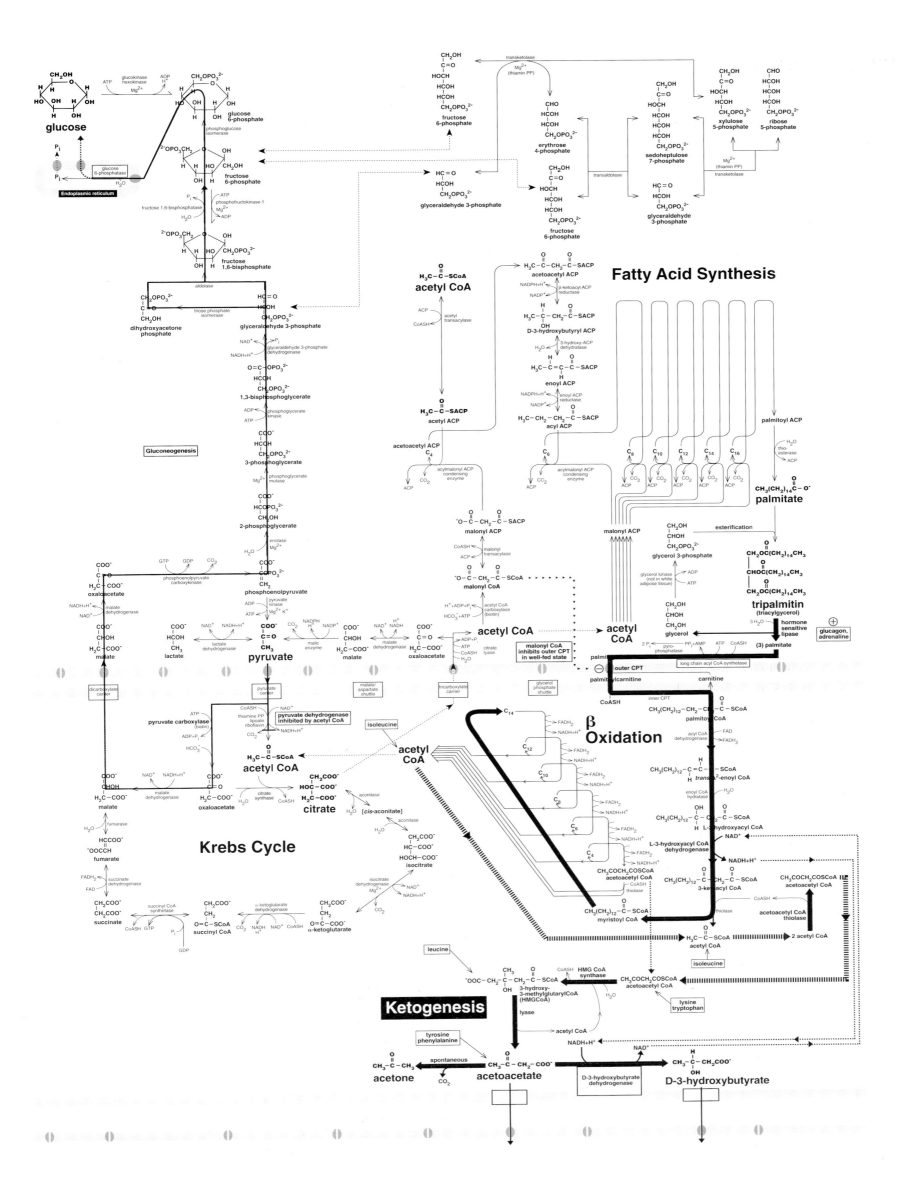

Fatty Acid Synthesis

β Oxidation

Krebs Cycle

Gluconeogenesis

Ketogenesis

Ketone body utilization

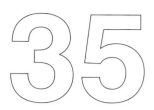
Chart 35 opposite. Ketone utilization.

The ketone bodies are an important fuel for the brain during starvation

The brain has an enormous need for respiratory fuel, each day requiring approximately 140g of glucose, which is equivalent to nearly 600 kcal (it should be remembered that brain cannot use fatty acids as a fuel). The large quantities of ATP produced are needed by the sodium pump mechanism which maintains the membrane potentials, which in turn are essential for the conduction of nerve impulses. Clearly, to stay alive, the brain must be supplied with respiratory fuel at all times!

During starvation, once the glycogen reserves are exhausted, the rate at which ketone bodies are produced from fatty acids by the liver is increased so they can be used by tissues, but particularly the brain, to generate ATP. Consequently, the use of glucose as a fuel by the brain is considerably reduced. The advantage of switching to the ketone bodies for energy is because, during starvation, glucose is obtained by gluconeogenesis from muscle protein. This causes wasting of the muscles and so the 'glucose-sparing' effect of the ketone bodies is an important adaptation to the stress of starvation.

Chart 35: Utilization of ketone bodies

The ketone bodies are first converted to acetyl CoA, which can then be oxidized by the Krebs cycle. The enzymes needed are **D-3-hydroxybutyrate dehydrogenase, 3-ketoacyl CoA transferase** and **acetoacetyl CoA thiolase**. It should be noted that the 3-ketoacyl CoA transferase is not found in liver. Consequently, the liver is unable to use the ketone bodies as respiratory fuel. On the other hand, although several tissues are capable of ketone utilization — notably muscle and kidney — they are particularly important as a fuel for brain and other nerve cells during starvation.

As illustrated in the chart opposite, D-3-hydroxybutyrate dehydrogenase is bound to the inner mitochondrial membrane, where it catalyses the formation of acetoacetate from D-3-hydroxybutyrate. Then, in the presence of 3-ketoacyl-CoA transferase, CoA is transferred from succinyl CoA to form acetoacetyl CoA. Subsequently, in the presence of CoA and acetoacetyl CoA thiolase, acetoacetyl CoA is cleaved to yield two molecules of acetyl CoA for oxidation in the Krebs cycle.

ATP yield from the complete oxidation of D-3-hydroxybutyrate

The oxidation of D-3-hydroxybutyrate generates two molecules of acetyl CoA which yield a net total of 26 molecules of ATP as follows:

	ATP yield
D-3-hydroxybutyrate dehydrogenase	
1 NADH+H$^+$	3
Krebs cycle	
6 NADH+H$^+$	18
2 FADH$_2$	4
Succinyl CoA synthetase (via GTP)	1
	26

Similarly, acetoacetate can generate a total of 23 molecules of ATP.

It should be noted that one of the pair of succinyl CoA molecules is temporarily diverted from Krebs cycle for the 3-ketoacyl CoA transferase reaction, where it 'activates' acetoacetate. This energy is therefore not available for ATP synthesis. The succinate liberated is, however, free to return to Krebs cycle for further oxidation.

In comparison with glucose, the ketone bodies are a very good respiratory fuel. Whereas 100g of glucose generates 10.7kg of ATP, 100g of D-3-hydroxybutyric acid can yield 12.7kg ATP, and 100g of acetoacetic acid produces 11.4kg of ATP.

Diagram 35.1. A generalized scheme representing the delivery of glucose and ketone bodies to nerve cells
The diagram shows the relationship of a capillary to a non-myelinated and a myelinated axon. Electron microscopy has demonstrated that, in myelinated axons, small clusters of mitochondria occur at the node of Ranvier. It is most probable that in myelinated axons the glucose transporters will also be located at these nodes, which are very metabolically active. On the other hand, in non-myelinated axons, mitochondria and glucose transporters are probably distributed uniformly along the length of the axon.

In both types of axon, glucose and the ketone bodies diffuse from the capillary, through the axolemma (via the Glu T3 glucose transporter) and into the axoplasm for metabolism.

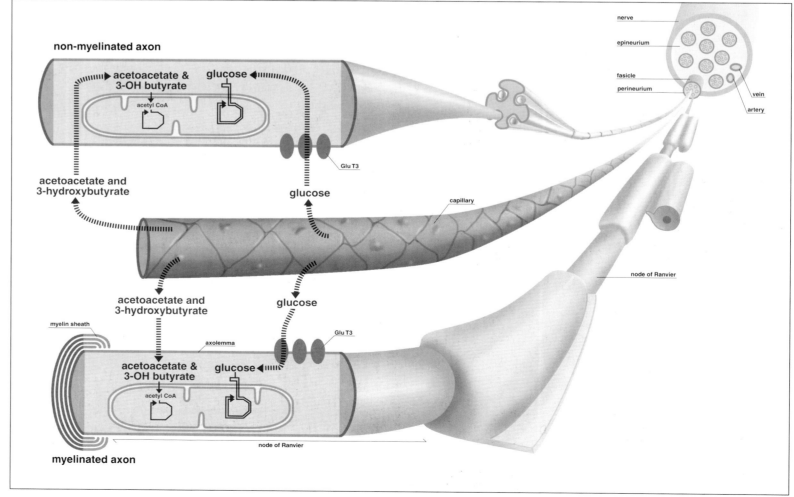

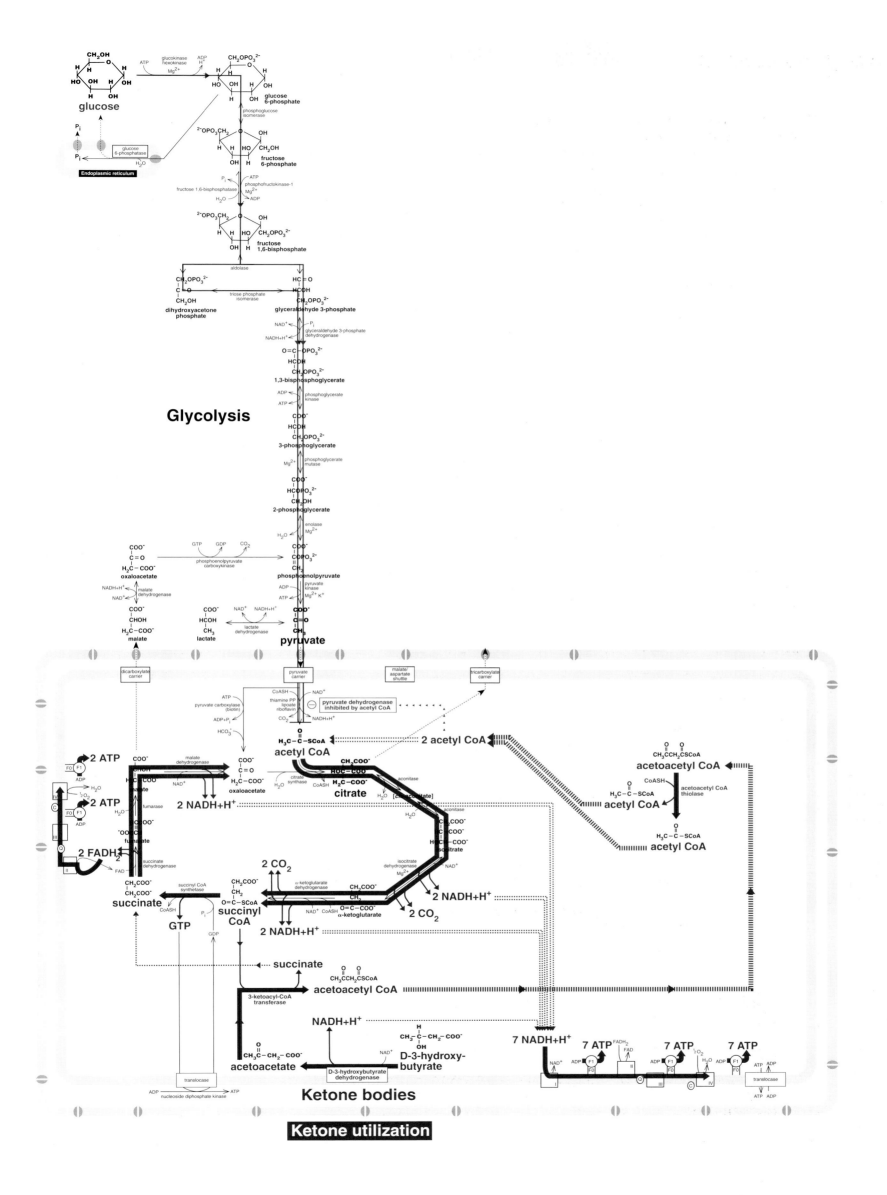

Glycolysis

Ketone bodies

β-Oxidation of unsaturated fatty acids

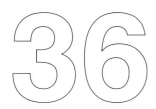

Chart 36 opposite. β-Oxidation of linoleic acid ($C_{18:2}$ n-6).

The naturally occurring unsaturated fatty acids have double bonds in the *cis*-configuration, but β-oxidation, as described in Chapter 15, produces intermediates with the *trans*- configuration. This stereoisomeric complication means that β-oxidation of unsaturated fatty acids requires two additional enzymes: **3,2-enoyl CoA isomerase**, and **2,4-dienoyl reductase**.

Chart 36: β-Oxidation of linoleic acid

The β-oxidation of the polyunsaturated fatty acid, linoleic acid, is illustrated in Chart 36, which demonstrates the similarities and differences in comparison to the saturated fatty acid derivative, palmitoyl CoA.

Cycles 1–3

The first three cycles of β-oxidation whereby linoleate ($C_{18:2}$) is shortened to dodecadienoate ($C_{12:2}$) (via $C_{16:2}$ and $C_{14:2}$), are identical to the reactions for saturated fatty acids described in Chapter 15.

Cycle 4 requires 3,2-enoyl CoA isomerase, (*cis*-Δ^3 [or *trans*-Δ^3]→*trans*-Δ^2-enoyl CoA isomerase)

The all *cis*-$C_{12:2}$ product (*cis*-Δ^3, *cis*-Δ^6-dodecadienoyl CoA, is not a substrate for enoyl CoA hydratase. The enzyme 3,2-enoyl CoA isomerase catalyses conversion of the *cis*-Δ^3 double bond to a *trans*-Δ^2 double bond. The hydration of the resulting *trans*-Δ^2-enoyl CoA is mediated by enoyl CoA hydratase. The dehydrogenase and thiolase reactions subsequently produce ($C_{10:1}$) decenoyl CoA and acetyl CoA.

Cycle 5 requires both a 'novel' reductase and the isomerase

Cycle 5 begins with ($C_{10:1}$) *cis*-Δ^4-decenoyl CoA, which is oxidized as usual by acyl CoA dehydrogenase. However, the *cis*-Δ^4 double bond of the *trans*-Δ^2, *cis*-Δ^4 product inhibits the hydratase reaction. A recently discovered enzyme, **2,4-dienoyl reductase**, catalyses the reduction of this metabolite by NADPH+H^+ to form the *trans*-Δ^3-enoyl CoA intermediate. This is then isomerized by the versatile 3,2-isomerase which changes the *trans*-Δ^3- to the *trans*-Δ^2- enoyl CoA form, which is a substrate for enoyl CoA hydratase. The usual sequence of β-oxidation reactions catalysed by the dehydrogenase and thiolase then produce ($C_{8:0}$) octanoyl CoA.

Cycles 6–8

Since ($C_{8:0}$) octanoyl CoA is fully saturated, it is oxidized by the familiar β-oxidation pathway to yield acetyl CoA.

What about the epimerase reaction?

Several textbooks describe the need for a '3-hydroxyacyl CoA epimerase' in the pathway for the β-oxidation of unsaturated fatty acids. This is because it used to be thought that enoyl CoA hydratase added water across a *cis*-Δ^2 double bond to form the D-isomer of hydroxyacyl CoA, i.e. not the L-isomer needed for 3-L-hydroxyacyl CoA dehydrogenase. The epimerase was thought to be needed to invert the configuration of the hydroxyl group at C_3 from the D-isomer to the L-isomer, thereby providing a suitable substrate for the 3-L-hydroxyacyl CoA dehydrogenase.

Current opinion is that the epimerase is not present in the mitochondria but is instead found in the peroxisomes. Indeed, there is evidence which suggests that this 'epimerase' activity is due to the reactions of two distinct 2-enoyl CoA hydratases which have been discovered recently in peroxisomes.

Fatty acid nomenclature

This is complicated and a knowledge of Greek helps. The various elements involved in the naming of fatty acids are summarized in Diagram 36.1.

Diagram 36.1. Fatty acid nomenclature. **NB**: Although the compounds shown could exist in theory, relatively few are known to occur in nature except as metabolic intermediates.

Number of carbon atoms present	**Prefix** C_6	C_8	C_{10}	C_{12}	C_{14}	C_{16}	C_{18}	C_{20}	C_{22}	C_{24}	C_{26}	**Suffix**
Number of carbon-to-carbon double-bonds present nil	hexan...	octan...	decan...	dodecan...	tetradecan...	hexadecan...	octadecan...	eicosan...	docosan...	tetracosan...	hexacosan...	...oic
1	hexen...	octen...	decen...	dodecen...	tetradecen...	hexadecen...	octadecen...	eicosen...	docosen...	tetracosen...	hexacosen...	...oic
2	hexa...	octa...	deca...	dodeca...	tetradeca...	hexadeca...	octadeca...	eicosa...	docosa...	tetracosa...	hexacosa...	...dienoic
3		octa...	deca...	dodeca...	tetradeca...	hexadeca...	octadeca...	eicosa...	docosa...	tetracosa...	hexacosa...	...trienoic
4			deca...	dodeca...	tetradeca...	hexadeca...	octadeca...	eicosa...	docosa...	tetracosa...	hexacosa...	...tetraenoic
5				dodeca...	tetradeca...	hexadeca...	octadeca...	eicosa...	docosa...	tetracosa...	hexacosa...	...pentaenoic
6					tetradeca...	hexadeca...	octadeca...	eicosa...	docosa...	tetracosa...	hexacosa...	...hexaenoic

Identification of carbon atoms

Numbering from carboxyl carbon atom	10	9	8	7	6	5	4	3	2	1
Greek letters	ω				ε	δ	γ	β	α	
Numbering from ω carbon atom	ω1	ω2	ω3	ω4	ω5	ω6				
Numbering from n carbon atom (methyl group)	n-1	n-2	n-3	n-4	n-5	n-6				

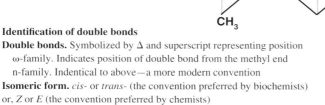 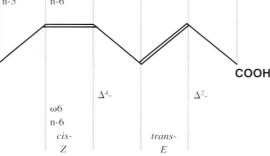

Identification of double bonds

Double bonds. Symbolized by Δ and superscript representing position
 ω-family. Indicates position of double bond from the methyl end
 n-family. Indentical to above—a more modern convention
Isomeric form. *cis*- or *trans*- (the convention preferred by biochemists)
or, *Z* or *E* (the convention preferred by chemists)

Δ^{4-} Δ^{2-}
ω6   n-6   *cis*   *trans*
Z   E

Summary

The fatty acid shown above is named as follows:
Length of carbon chain is **10** carbon atoms, C_{10}
There are two **2** carbon-to-carbon double-bonds present. $C_{10:2}$
Hence the above example is a $C_{10:2}$ unsaturated fatty acid, namely ***trans*-Δ^2-, *cis*-Δ^4-decadienoic acid**
which is a **n-6** (or alternatively **ω6**) unsaturated fatty acid.
NB: This is not a common, naturally occurring fatty acid. However, its thioester with CoA is formed during the β-oxidation of linoleic acid (see Chart opposite)

Confusion! The α- and γ- prefixes of α- and γ-linolenate are **not** based on the above conventions.

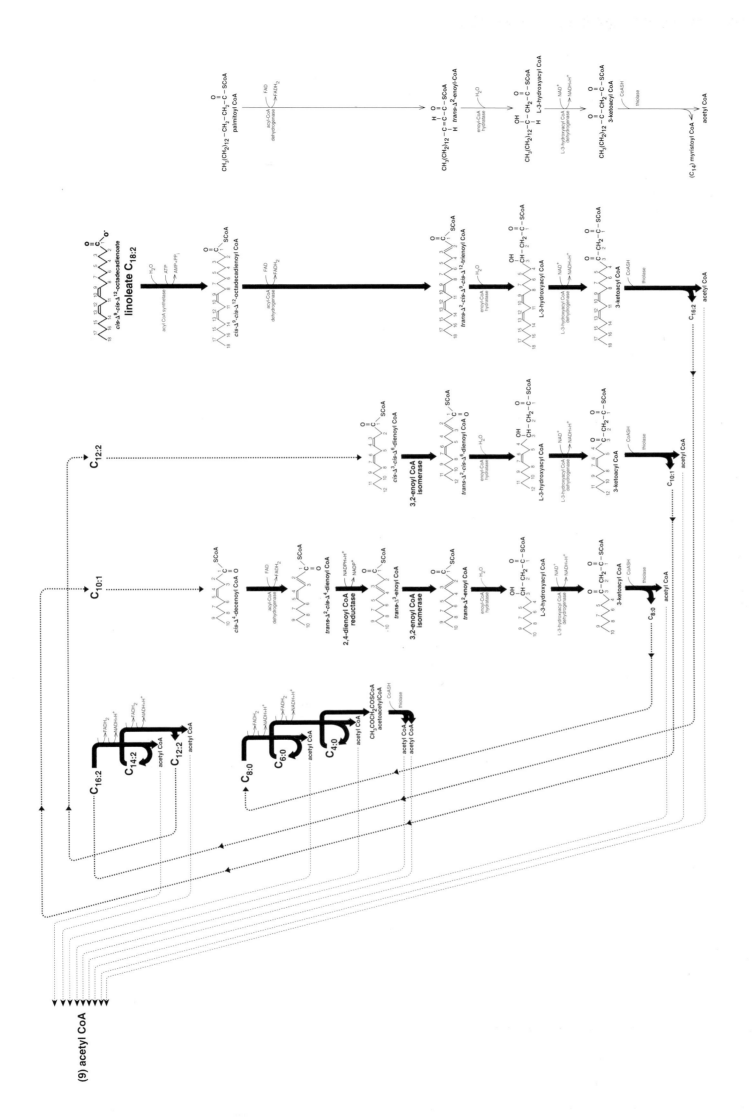

Peroxisomal β-oxidation

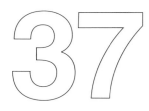

Chart 37 opposite. Peroxisomal β-oxidation of lignoceric acid.

Mitochondria are not the only location for β-oxidation

The pathway for the β-oxidation of fatty acids was once thought to be restricted exclusively to mitochondria. However, mammalian peroxisomal β-oxidation of fatty acids was confirmed in 1976 by Lazarow and de Duve. Peroxisomal β-oxidation occurs in both the liver and kidney. It is now thought that approximately 90% of short- and medium-chain length fatty acids are oxidized in the mitochondria, whilst approximately 10% are oxidized in the peroxisomes in the basal state. However under conditions of induced proliferation of the peroxisomes, whether by drugs (e.g. clofibrate) or a high-fat diet, the relative importance of peroxisomal β-oxidation is substantially increased.

Whereas the structural changes in the metabolic intermediates formed during β-oxidation are chemically identical in both the peroxisomes and mitochondria, different and distinct enzymes are involved in the two organelles. An important difference in peroxisomal β-oxidation is that it is much more versatile than the mitochondrial pathway. It is capable of metabolizing a wide variety of fatty acid analogues, notably dicarboxylic acids and prostaglandins. However, current opinion is that the main function of peroxisomal β-oxidation is for chain-shortening of very long-chain fatty acids (i.e. greater than C_{22} and longer) in preparation for their subsequent oxidation by mitochondria.

Chart 37: Chain-shortening of very long-chain fatty acids by peroxisomal β-oxidation

The distinguishing features of peroxisomal β-oxidation can be seen in the chart, using C_{24} lignoceroate as an example:

1 **Activation.** A **long-chain acyl CoA synthetase** which is located on the cytosolic side of the peroxisomal membrane activates the fatty acid to form **lignoceroyl CoA**.

2 **Transport across peroxisomal membrane.** The peroxisomal membrane contains a non-specific, **pore-forming protein** which enables the lignoceroyl CoA to diffuse across it by passive transport. It also allows the products of β-oxidation to diffuse out of the peroxisome.

3 **Oxidation of fatty acids.** In peroxisomes, the first oxidation step is catal-ysed by the FAD-containing enzyme **acyl CoA oxidase**. **NB:** This reaction, in which the electrons are passed directly to oxygen, is insensitive to the respiratory chain inhibitor, cyanide (see Chapter 3). The hydrogen peroxide formed is broken down to water and oxygen in the presence of **catalase**. Note also that in contrast to mitochondrial β-oxidation, which employs FAD-dependent acyl CoA dehydrogenase, ATP is not formed in peroxisomes at this stage and instead the energy is dissipated as heat.

4 **Bifunctional enzyme.** The bifunctional enzyme has both **enoyl CoA hydratase** and **L-3-hydroxyacyl CoA dehydrogenase** activity. The dehydrogenase forms NADH+H[+], the accumulation of which could become rate-limiting. The fate of NADH+H[+] depends on the energy status of the cell. It could in theory pass into the mitochondrion via the malate–aspartate shuttle. Alternatively, evidence using isolated rat liver peroxisomes suggests that the **lactate dehydrogenase** reaction could be important for the reoxidation of NADH+H[+], as shown in the chart.

5 **The products of peroxisomal β-oxidation.** The products of chain shortening are **acetyl CoA** and the newly formed acyl CoA (i.e. palmitoyl CoA, as shown in Chart 37). The precise details of their subsequent fate are not yet clear. In principle, both of these could leave the peroxisome unchanged, or they could be hydrolysed by peroxisomal hydrolase to acetate, or to their free acyl derivatives. Another possibility is that acylcarnitine might be formed in the peroxisome prior to export to the mitochondria for further β-oxidation. Because of this uncertainty, the representation in the chart should be regarded as a simplification.

Peroxisomal β-oxidation of unsaturated fatty acids and the 'trifunctional' enzyme

The mitochondrial β-oxidation of unsaturated fatty acids is described in Chapter 36. However, there is now evidence which suggests that some unsaturated fatty acids are readily metabolized by peroxisomal β-oxidation. Accordingly, peroxisomes have a 2,4-dienoyl CoA reductase. They also have 3,2-enoyl CoA isomerase activity. Indeed, there is evidence to suggest that the latter is associated with the 'bifunctional' enzyme, thereby conferring upon it 'trifunctional' status.

Saturated

Notional name	Systematic name	Common name	
$C_{6:0}$	hexanoic acid	caproic acid	Latin *caper* goat
$C_{8:0}$	octanoic acid	caprylic acid	Latin *caper* goat
$C_{10:0}$	decanoic acid	capric acid	Found in butter, coconut oil etc
$C_{12:0}$	dodecanoic acid	lauric acid	Found in berries of laurel
$C_{14:0}$	tetradecanoic acid	myristic acid	*Myristica*: nutmeg tree (found in nutmeg oil etc.)
$C_{16:0}$	hexadecanoic acid	palmitic acid	Found in palm oil
$C_{18:0}$	octadecanoic acid	stearic acid	Greek *stear* fat
$C_{20:0}$	eicosanoic acid	arachidic acid	*Arachis*: peanut
$C_{22:0}$	docosanoic acid	behenic acid	In oil of ben, seed oil of the horse-radish tree, *Moringa pterygospermum*
$C_{24:0}$	tetracosanoic acid	lignoceric acid	Latin *lignum* wood (found in beech-wood tar)
$C_{26:0}$	hexacosanoic acid	cerotic acid	Greek *keros* wax
$C_{28:0}$	octacosanoic acid	montanic acid	In montan wax (extracted from lignite)

Unsaturated

Notional name	Systematic name	Common name	
$C_{4:1}$	*trans*-Δ^2-tetraenoic acid	crotonic acid	Greek *kroton* castor-oil plant.
$C_{16:1}$n-7	*cis*-Δ^9-hexadecenoic acid	palmitoleic acid	Palm oil
$C_{18:1}$n-9	*cis*-Δ^9-octadecenoic acid	oleic acid	Latin *oleum* oil
$C_{18:1}$n-7	*cis*-Δ^{11}-octadecenoic acid	vaccenic acid	Latin *vacca* cow (in beef fat)
$C_{18:2}$n-6	all *cis*-$\Delta^{9,12}$-octadecadienoate	linoleic acid	Latin *linum* flax, and *oleum* oil (in linseed oil etc)
$C_{18:3}$n-3	all *cis*-$\Delta^{9,12,15}$-octadecatrienoic acid	α-linolenic acid	
$C_{18:3}$n-6	all *cis*-$\Delta^{6,9,12}$-octadecatrienoic acid	GLA (γ-linolenic acid)	GLA (Found in evening primrose oil)
$C_{20:1}$n-9	*cis*-Δ^{11}-eicosenoic acid	gondoic acid	
$C_{20:4}$n-6	all *cis*-$\Delta^{5,8,11,14}$-eicosatetraenoic acid	arachidonic acid	*Arachis*: peanut
$C_{20:5}$n-3	all *cis*-$\Delta^{5,8,11,14,17}$-eicosa-pentaenoic acid	EPA (timnodonic acid)	Eicosa Pentaenoic Acid (found in fish oil)
$C_{22:1}$n-9	*cis*-Δ^{13}-docosenoic acid	erucic acid	Latin *eruca* cabbage (in seed oil of *Cruciferae*: mustard, rape etc.)
$C_{22:5}$n-3	all *cis*-$\Delta^{7,10,13,16,19}$-docosa-pentaenoic acid	clupanodonic acid	*Clupeidae* herring (found in fish oil)
$C_{22:6}$n-3	all *cis*-$\Delta^{4,7,10,13,16,19}$-docosa-hexaenoic acid	DHA (cervonic acid)	Docosa Hexaenoic Acid (found in fish oil)

Diagram 37.1. Nomenclature of some naturally occurring fatty acids.

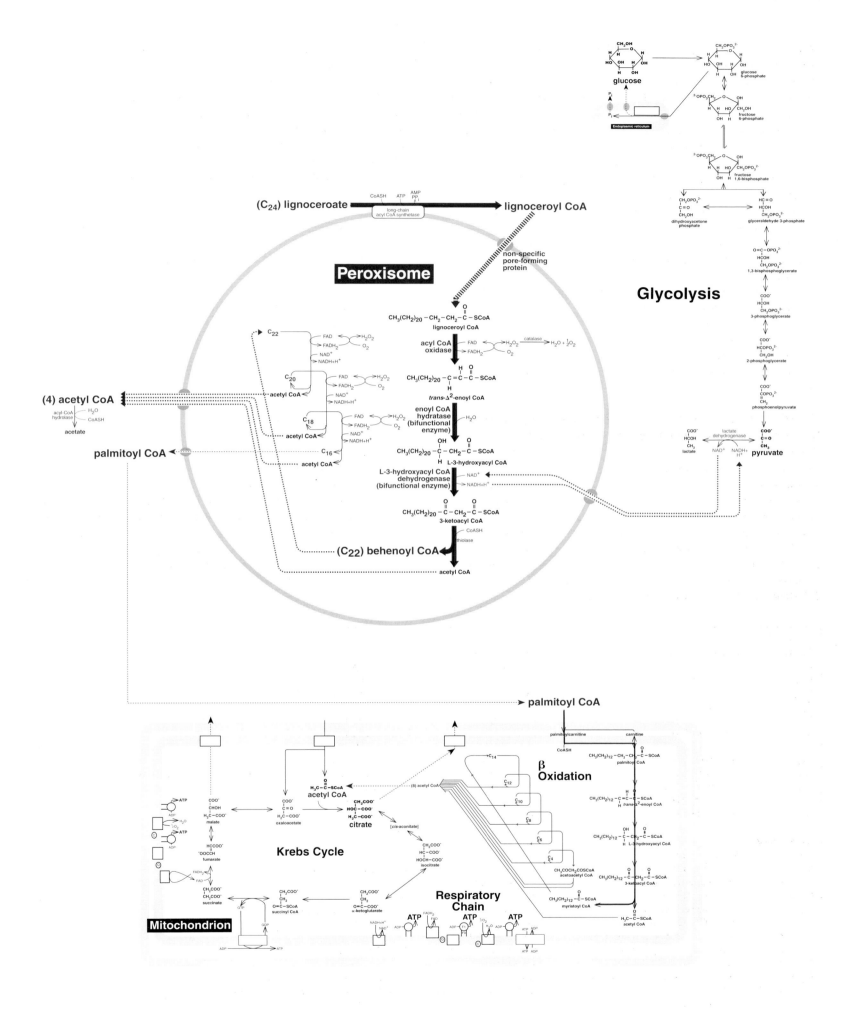

Elongation and desaturation of fatty acids

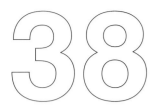

We have seen in Chapter 11 how $(C_{16:0})$ palmitate, and $(C_{18:0})$ stearate, are formed by the fatty acid synthase complex. These products can be modified in various ways. Additional carbon atoms can be added to form long-chain fatty acids. Alternatively, or as well, fatty acids can be desaturated to yield products with one or more double bonds. The long-chain polyunsaturated fatty acids so formed are used for synthesizing membrane phospholipids and the prostaglandins.

Chart 38 opposite. Elongation and desaturation of fatty acids.

Elongation of fatty acids by the endoplasmic reticulum pathway

An example of chain elongation followed by desaturation is shown in the chart opposite. Here $(C_{18:3})$ **γ-linolenic acid** is initially lengthened to $(C_{20:3})$ **dihomo-γ-linolenoyl CoA**, which is desaturated to $(C_{20:4})$ **arachidonoyl CoA**.

The endoplasmic reticulum pathway by which fatty acids are elongated is similar to the pathway for fatty acid synthesis described in Chapter 11. The principal differences are:
1 For chain elongation, the two NADPH+H⁺-dependent **reductase** enzymes and the **dehydratase** are located on the cytosolic surface of the smooth endoplasmic reticulum.
2 Instead of acyl carrier protein (ACP), the intermediates for chain elongation are bound to CoA.
3 The 2-carbon donor is **malonyl CoA** (not malonyl-ACP).

Desaturation of fatty acids

Mammals have four desaturases: Δ^4-, Δ^5-, Δ^6- and Δ^9-fatty acyl CoA desaturases. These enzymes have a broad chain-length specificity and occur mainly in liver.

A wide range of different fatty acids can be produced by a combination of the elongation and desaturase reactions. For example, in the chart opposite, **Δ^5-desaturase** is used to form arachidonic acid, whereas in Diagram 38.1, the **Δ^9-desaturase** is shown oxidizing $(C_{16:0})$ palmitoyl CoA to $(C_{16:1})$ palmitoleoyl CoA.

The desaturase system, which is located in the membrane of the smooth endoplasmic reticulum, consists of the **desaturase(s)**, **cytochrome b_5** and **cytochrome b_5 reductase.**

Diagram 38.1: The desaturation of palmitoyl CoA to form palmitoleoyl CoA

Diagram 38.1. The desaturation of palmitoyl CoA to form palmitoleoyl CoA.

The diagram illustrates the desaturation of palmitoyl CoA to palmitoleoyl CoA. It should be noted that molecular oxygen is the terminal electron acceptor and that it receives **two** pairs of electrons: one originating from the 9,10 double bond of palmitoyl CoA and the second donated by NADH+H⁺.

Let us first consider the electrons derived from the 9,10 C−H bonds of palmitoyl CoA in the reaction catalysed by **Δ^9-desaturase**. The desaturases are enzymes which contain non-haem ferric iron (Fe^{3+}). The electrons reduce two atoms of this to the ferrous (Fe^{2+}) state prior to the electrons being passed on to oxygen, which combines with $2H^+$ to form water.

Next consider the electrons provided by NADH+H⁺. A pair of electrons is donated to the FAD prosthetic group of **cytochrome b_5 reductase**, which is consequently reduced to $FADH_2$. The electrons are then accepted by **cytochrome b_5**, which in turn donates the electrons to oxygen, which combines with $2H^+$ to form water.

Elongation of short-chain fatty acids occurs in mitochondria

The mitochondrial pathway for chain elongation is essentially a reversal of β-oxidation with one exception. The last step in elongation, i.e. the reaction catalysed by **enoyl CoA reductase**, requires NADPH+H⁺ for elongation, whereas the corresponding enzyme for β-oxidation, acyl CoA dehydrogenase, requires FAD (Chart 38). The mitochondrial pathway appears to be important for elongating fatty acids containing 14, or fewer, carbon atoms. In the chart opposite, this is exemplified by the elongation of $(C_{14:0})$ myristoyl CoA to form $(C_{16:0})$ palmitoyl CoA.

Essential fatty acids

As mentioned earlier, higher mammals, including humans, have enzymes capable of desaturating fatty acids at the Δ^4-, Δ^5-, Δ^6- and Δ^9- positions. However, they are incapable of desaturation beyond the C_9 carbon atom. Nevertheless, certain polyunsaturated fatty acids are vital for maintaining health, in particular the 'n-6 family' members, dihomo-γ-linolenic acid and arachidonic acid. These are 20-carbon-atom chain-length fatty acids which are precursors of the eicosanoid hormones (Greek *eikosi*, twenty), i.e. the prostaglandins, thromboxanes and leukotrienes, which contain 20 carbon atoms. Accordingly, the 'n-6 family' precursor linoleic acid ($C_{18:2}$, all *cis*-$\Delta^{9,12}$), for example, is essential in the diet and is known as an 'essential fatty acid'. After sequential Δ^6-desaturation, 2-carbon chain-elongation, and Δ^5-desaturation, linoleic acid is transformed to arachidonic acid.

Evening primrose oil: 'the elixir of life'?

Normally, given a healthy diet, linoleic acid is an adequate precursor of its family of polyunsaturated fatty acids. There are circumstances, however, possibly including diabetes mellitus, where Δ^6-desaturase activity is relatively inactive, which limits the conversion of linoleic acid to dihomo-γ-linolenic acid and arachidonic acid. Evidence suggests that dietary supplementation with γ-linolenic acid ($C_{18:3}$, all *cis*-$\Delta^{6,9,12}$) is beneficial in preventing and minimizing many of the complications of diabetes. Indeed, evening primrose oil, which is rich in γ-linolenic acid, is currently enjoying a reputation for a wide range of health benefits. As illustrated in Chart 38 opposite, γ-linolenic acid is independent of Δ^6-desaturase to form the polyunsaturated products, since it requires only elongation and Δ^5-desaturation.

Therapeutic benefits of evening primrose oil and fish oils

The γ-linolenic acid in evening primrose oil is, via dihomo-γ-linolenic acid, a precursor of the series 1 prostaglandins. Fish oils are rich in the n-3 fatty acid eicosapentanoic acid, which is a precursor of the prostaglandin 3 series. It is known that out of the different prostaglandins, the series 2 prostaglandins have the most potent inflammatory effects, sometimes with pathological consequences. Dietary supplementation with γ-linolenic acid or eicosapentanoic acid causes proportionally enhanced production of the benign series 1 and 3 prostaglandins, thereby displacing the potent inflammatory effects of the 2 series. Clinical trials with these oils have shown beneficial effects in the treatment of inflammatory diseases such as psoriasis and rheumatoid arthritis.

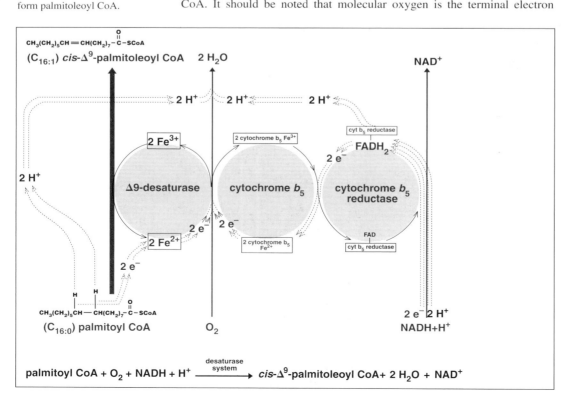

$CH_3(CH_2)_5CH = CH(CH_2)_7 - \overset{O}{\overset{\|}{C}} - SCoA$
$(C_{16:1})$ *cis*-Δ^9-palmitoleoyl CoA   2 H_2O NAD⁺

2 H⁺   2 H⁺   2 H⁺

2 Fe³⁺   2 cytochrome b_5 Fe³⁺   cyt b_5 reductase

FADH₂
2 e⁻

2 H⁺

Δ9-desaturase   cytochrome b_5 cytochrome b_5 reductase

2 Fe²⁺   2 e⁻   2 e⁻   2 cytochrome b_5 Fe²⁺

FAD
cyt b_5 reductase

2 e⁻

$CH_3(CH_2)_5CH - CH(CH_2)_7 - \overset{O}{\overset{\|}{C}} - SCoA$
$(C_{16:0})$ palmitoyl CoA O_2 2 e⁻ 2 H⁺
NADH+H⁺

palmitoyl CoA + O_2 + NADH + H⁺ $\xrightarrow{\text{desaturase system}}$ *cis*-Δ^9-palmitoleoyl CoA+ 2 H_2O + NAD⁺

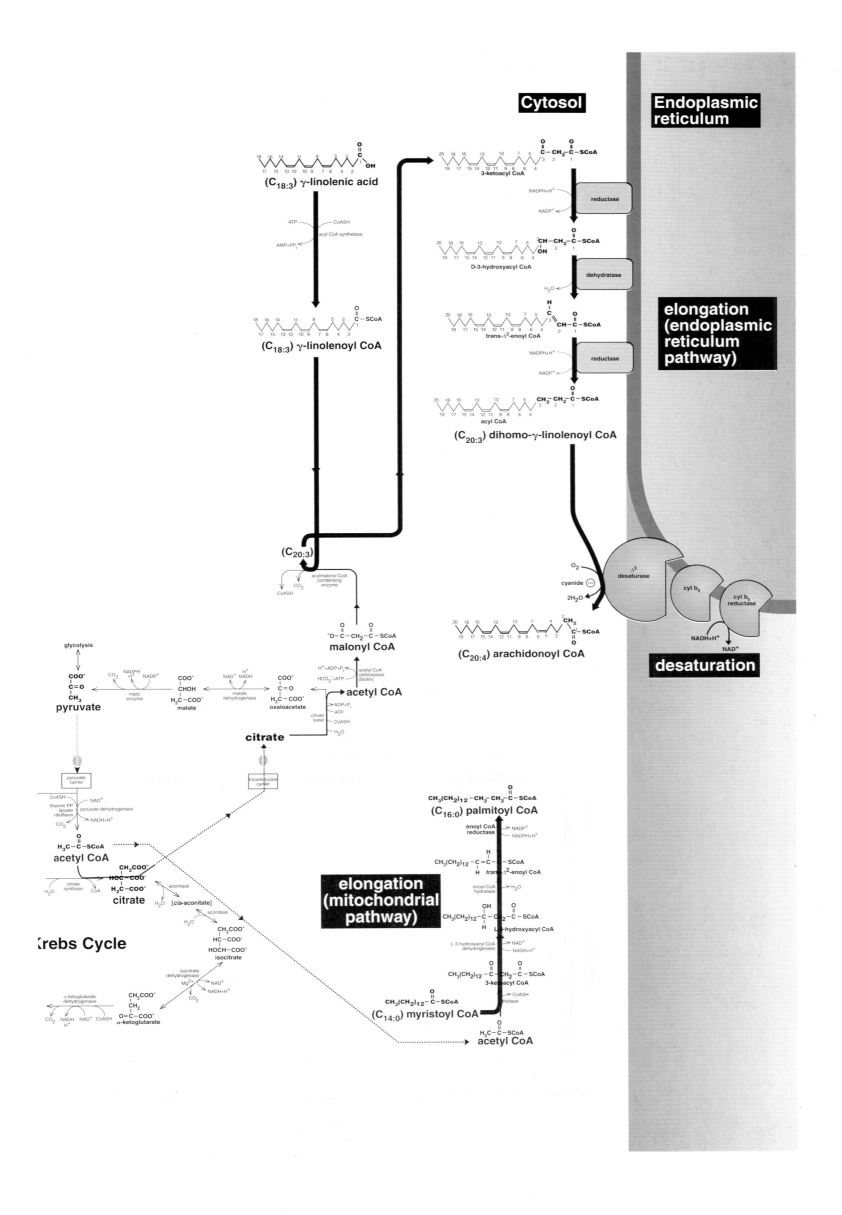

85

Metabolism of ethanol

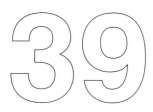

Alcohol, or more precisely ethanol, is a popular mood-altering compound which has been consumed over the centuries as wine, beer and, more recently, as spirits. Whereas there is evidence that suggests that the intake of small quantities of ethanol with food can be beneficial, excessive consumption can cause cirrhosis of the liver, or metabolic disturbances including fatty liver and hypoglycaemia.

Ethanol is metabolized by three enzyme systems

Chart 39 opposite. Metabolism of ethanol.

Ethanol is rapidly oxidized in the liver by three enzyme systems, but the relative physiological importance of these is not clear (see Diagram 39.1 and Chart 39). All three systems produce acetaldehyde, which is normally oxidized rapidly to acetate. Evidence suggests that the accumulation of acetaldehyde may be responsible for some of the unpleasant effects caused by drinking alcohol, e.g. the flushing which is often seen in those people (45% of Japanese and Chinese) who are genetically deficient in aldehyde dehydrogenase.

Alcohol dehydrogenase in the cytosol

There may be up to 20 different isoenzymes of alcohol dehydrogenase. The rate of this pathway is largely regulated by the availability of NAD^+. This in turn depends on the ability of the malate/aspartate shuttle (see Chapter 4) to transport reducing equivalents into the mitochondrion, and moreover on the ability of the respiratory chain to oxidize $NADH+H^+$ to NAD^+.

Microsomal ethanol-oxidizing system, MEOS

This system is located in the smooth endoplasmic reticulum and involves a cytochrome P450 enzyme. These are a family of monooxygenases concerned with the detoxication of ingested drugs and xenobiotics.

Peroxisomal oxidation of ethanol

Catalase uses hydrogen peroxide to oxidize alcohols such as methanol and ethanol to their corresponding aldehydes.

Metabolism of acetaldehyde

The acetaldehyde formed by any of the three systems mentioned above must now enter the mitochondrion for further oxidation by aldehyde dehydrogenase to form acetate. Finally this acetate could theoretically be activated to acetyl CoA for oxidation by Krebs cycle. However, in liver, the Krebs cycle is unable to oxidize this acetyl CoA, as we will see below, because of the prevailing high ratio of $NADH+H^+/NAD^+$ in the mitochondrial matrix. Consequently the acetate will probably leave the liver for oxidation by the extrahepatic tissues.

The biochemical effects of ethanol
Increased $NADH+H^+/NAD^+$ ratio

Following ingestion of ethanol, the cytosolic **alcohol dehydrogenase** reaction and the mitochondrial **aldehyde dehydrogenase** reaction both produce $NADH+H^+$, with relative depletion of NAD^+ so that the ratio of $NADH+H^+/NAD^+$ is significantly increased. This has the following effects:

1 Gluconeogenesis is inhibited. As shown in the chart opposite, the high $NADH+H^+/NAD^+$ ratio in the cytosol displaces the equilibrium of the dehydrogenase reactions in favour of the reduced reactant. In particular, **pyruvate** is reduced to **lactate**, and **oxaloacetate** is reduced to **malate**, thereby preventing the flow of metabolites in the direction of gluconeogenesis. This can cause hypoglycaemia (see below).

2 Krebs cycle is inhibited in liver. The high $NADH+H^+/NAD^+$ ratio in the mitochondrial matrix prevents the oxidation of **isocitrate** to **α-ketoglutarate**, of **α-ketoglutarate** to **succinyl CoA**, and of **malate** to **oxaloacetate**. Consequently, although acetate can be activated to acetyl CoA for metabolism in the liver, it is more likely that acetate will be exported for metabolism by the extrahepatic tissues.

Hyperlactataemia and gout

The accumulation of lactate results in hyperlactataemia. This can cause hyperuricaemia because lactate and urate share, and so compete for, the same mechanism for renal tubular secretion. Gout occurs when uric acid, which is sparingly soluble in plasma, crystallizes in the joints, particularly the toes.

Ethanol interactions with drugs

Long-term treatment with many drugs, for example the barbiturates, causes proliferation of the smooth endoplasmic reticulum and increases the activity of the cytochrome P450 isoenzymes involved in their metabolism and clearance from the body. Similarly, chronic ingestion of excessive quantities of ethanol causes increased proliferation of the endoplasmic reticulum and induction of these enzymes. This means that a sober alcoholic patient will metabolize and inactivate these drugs very rapidly and may need higher than normal doses for treatment. However, in the drunken alcoholic, ethanol preferentially competes with these drugs for metabolism by the cytochrome P450 isoenzymes. As a result, the inactivation and clearance of the barbiturates is suppressed, with the risk of lethal consequences.

Ethanol-induced fasting hypoglycaemia

This condition develops in chronically malnourished individuals several hours after a heavy drinking binge. This is caused by the inhibition of gluconeogenesis, as described above.

Diagram 39.1. The three enzyme systems responsible for ethanol metabolism.

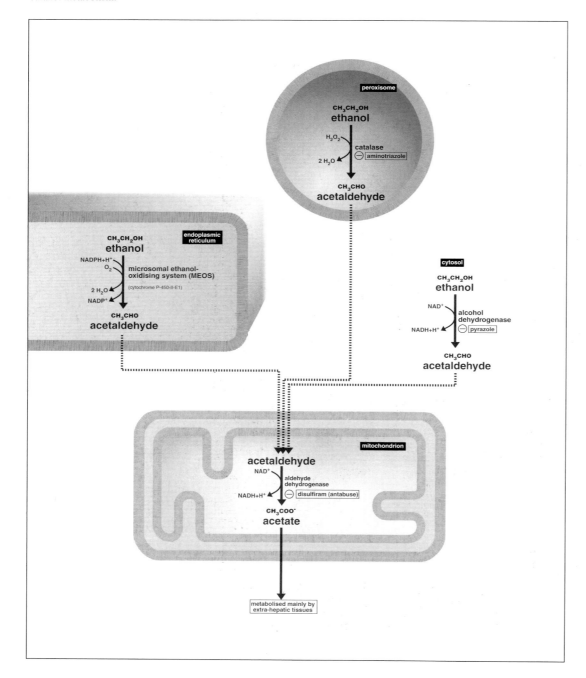

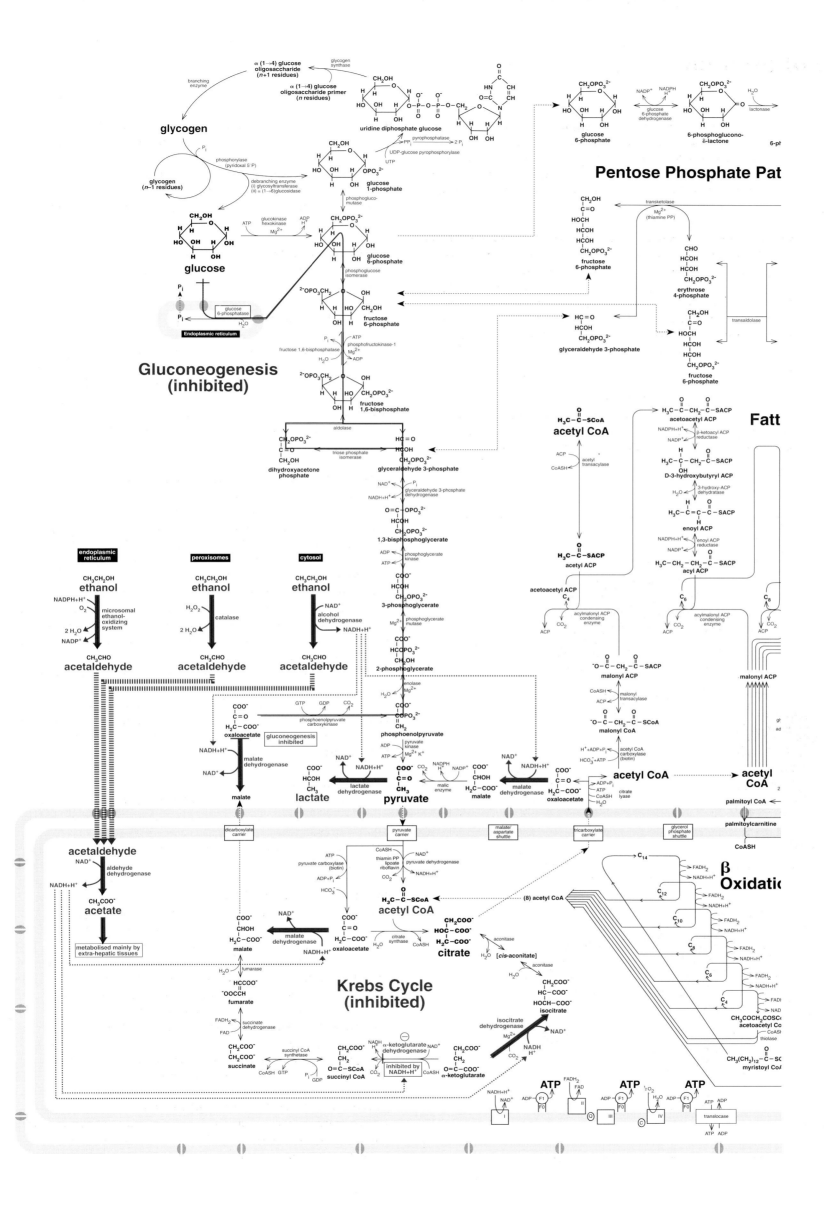

Sorbitol, galactitol, glucuronate and xylitol

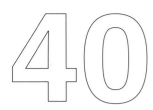

Chart 40.1: Sorbitol, the dietary (exogenous) friend but endogenous foe
Dietary sorbitol as a food sweetener

Sorbitol is a sugar alcohol which is used as a food sweetener in diabetic diets, and has a sweetness value which is approximately 50% of that of sucrose. Patients with diabetes can eat small quantities of sorbitol safely because it is transported relatively slowly across cell membranes, and is absorbed slowly from the intestines.

Chart 40.1 opposite top. Sorbitol metabolism.

Chart 40.3 opposite bottom. Glucuronate and xylitol metabolism.

Endogenously produced sorbitol and cataracts. 'the polyol-osmotic theory for the formation of diabetic cataracts'

Although the poor ability of extracellular sorbitol to cross cell membranes favours its use as a sweetener for diabetic food, paradoxically this property can also cause problems. This is because sorbitol produced **endogenously** within cells such as neurons and the optical lens, accumulates within the cell and is metabolized very slowly. Under normal circumstances this is not a problem, since **aldose reductase**, the enzyme which converts glucose to sorbitol, has a K_m for glucose of 70 mmol/l. Hence, it is relatively inactive when the blood glucose concentration is within normal limits of around 3–6 mmol/l. However, in uncontrolled diabetes with glucose levels of 25 mmol/l or higher, sorbitol formation occurs at a greater rate, and elevated tissue sorbitol levels have been implicated with certain complications of diabetes such as neuropathy and cataracts. For example, *in vitro* studies have shown that if rabbit lenses are incubated in media containing very high glucose concentrations (35 mmol/l), they accumulate sorbitol. Consequently, the intralenticular osmotic pressure increases, causing the lens to swell and become opaque. This can be prevented by aldose reductase inhibitors such as sorbinil.

Sorbitol catabolism

Sorbitol is metabolized by **sorbitol dehydrogenase**, which is particularly active in liver, to form fructose in a reaction coupled to the formation of NADH+H⁺. This increases the cytosolic NADH+H⁺/NAD⁺ ratio, which both favours the reduction of dihydroxyacetone phosphate to glycerol 3-phosphate and inhibits glycolysis by favouring the reduction of 1,3-bis-

phosphoglycerate to glyceraldehyde 3-phosphate. Also, experiments with rat lens have demonstrated that, when the aldose reductase pathway is active, the sorbitol formed is metabolized by sorbitol dehydrogenase to form fructose, which is metabolized to **glycerol 3-phosphate**, since glycolysis is inhibited at the glyceraldehyde 3-phosphate dehydrogenase reaction. Finally, because aldose reductase generates NADP⁺, the pentose phosphate pathway is stimulated.

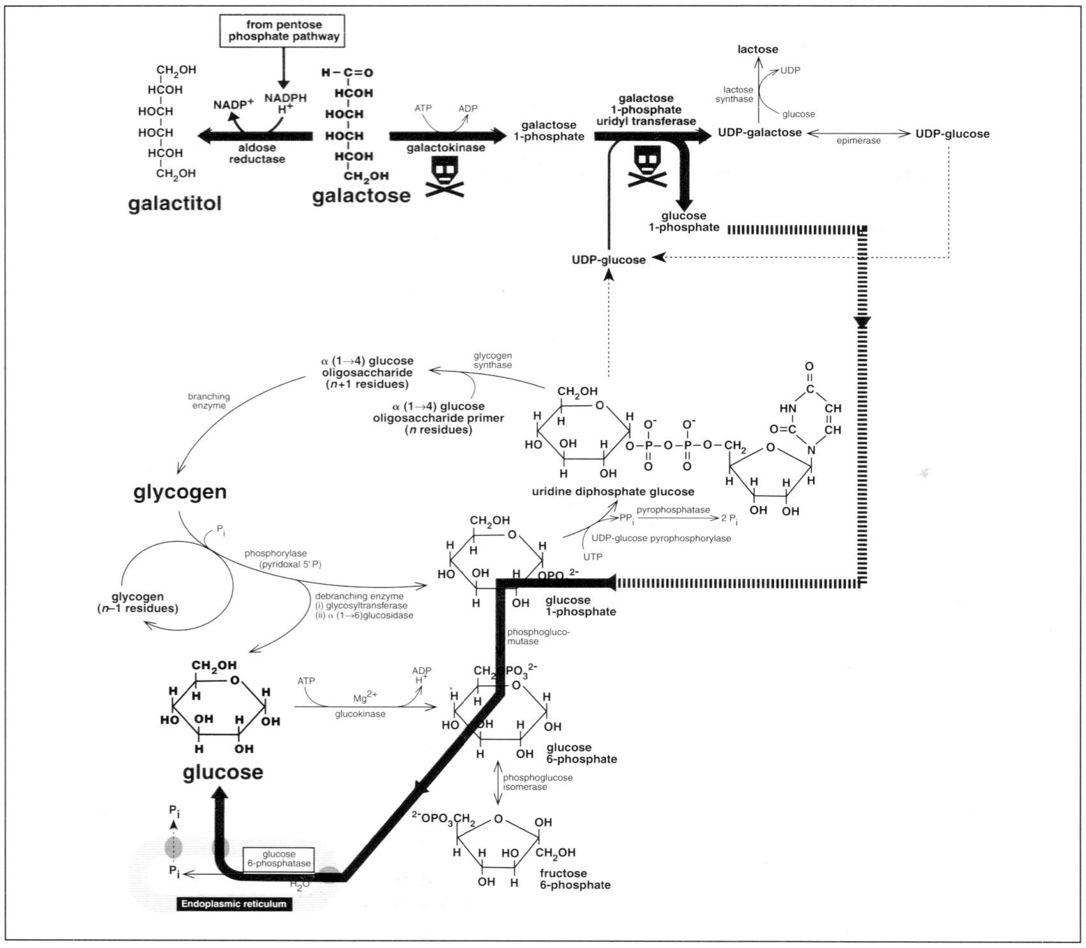

Chart 40.2: Galactose and galactitol metabolism
Uses of galactose

Galactose is used as a component of cerebrosides and glycoproteins, and during lactation is used to synthesize lactose. The major dietary source of galactose is lactose in milk. Hydrolysis of lactose by intestinal lactase yields glucose and galactose. Surplus galactose is metabolized to glucose as shown in Chart 40.2.

Inborn errors of galactose metabolism

Patients with galactosaemia caused either by galactokinase deficiency or by galactose 1-phosphate uridyltransferase deficiency have been described. In both conditions dietary galactose cannot be metabolized. Consequently, it accumulates in the blood and enters the cells of the lens, where it is reduced to **galactitol** by **aldose reductase**. It is believed that this can cause cataracts by a mechanism similar to that described for sorbitol.

Chart 40.3: Glucuronate and xylitol metabolism
Glucuronate conjugates with bilirubin, steroids and drug metabolites

Uridine diphosphate glucuronate (UDP glucuronate) is formed by oxidation of **UDP glucose** in the presence of UDP glucose dehydrogenase. Hydrophobic molecules such as bilirubin, steroid hormones and many drugs are conjugated with glucuronate by **UDP glucuronyl transferase** to form a water-soluble glucuronide derivative prior to urinary excretion by the kidney. In Crigler–Najjar sydrome, deficiency of UDP glucuronyl transferase causes increased levels of unconjugated bilirubin, which is bound to albumin, to accumulate in the blood. If the levels exceed the binding capacity of albumin, the unconjugated bilirubin will be taken up by the brain, causing kernicterus.

Glucuronate is the precursor of vitamin C, but not in humans

UDP glucuronate is metabolized to L-gulonate. In most animals (with the notable exception of humans, the other primates, the guinea-pig and the fruit bat), L-gulonate can be metabolized to ascorbate (vitamin C).

Metabolism of glucuronate and xylitol: the glucuronate/xylulose pathway

UDP Glucuronate is metabolized via the ketose, **L-xylulose** to **xylitol**. Xylitol is oxidized to D-xylulose which is phosphorylated to **xylulose 5-phosphate**, which enters the pentose phosphate pathway before joining the glycolytic (or gluconeogenic) pathway.

Inborn error of metabolism: essential pentosuria

This is a very rare benign condition, most frequently found in Jewish people, in which large quantities (up to 4 g per day) of L-xylulose are excreted in the urine. The condition is due to deficiency of **L-xylulose reductase**.

Xylitol in chewing gum prevents dental decay

Since the 1970s, there has been much interest in the use of xylitol as a sweetener, since it appears to have properties that limit dental caries. Clinical trials indicate that 7–10 g per day of xylitol in chewing gum can provide good resistance to dental decay in children. This cariostatic effect is thought to be due to both its ability to interfere with the metabolism of *Streptococcus mutans* (the organism in plaque responsible for caries) and also its ability to stabilize solutions of calcium phosphate, which favours remineralization of enamel.

Chart 40.2. Galactose and galactitol metabolism.

[Chart 40.2 diagram: Galactose and galactitol metabolism, showing pathways including galactitol, galactose, galactokinase, galactose 1-phosphate, galactose 1-phosphate uridyl transferase, UDP-galactose, UDP-glucose, lactose synthase, glucose 1-phosphate, glycogen, glucose, glucose 6-phosphate, fructose 6-phosphate, uridine diphosphate glucose, and associated enzymes within the endoplasmic reticulum.]

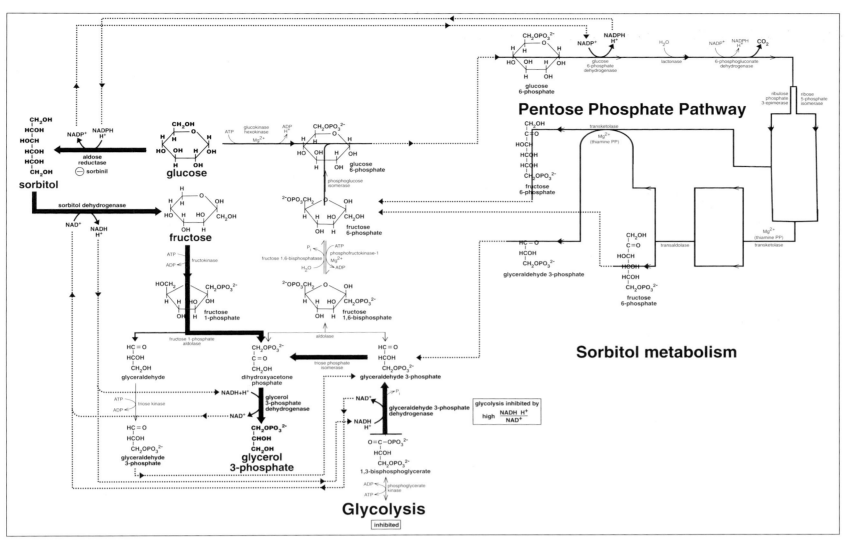

Pentose Phosphate Pathway

Sorbitol metabolism

Glycolysis

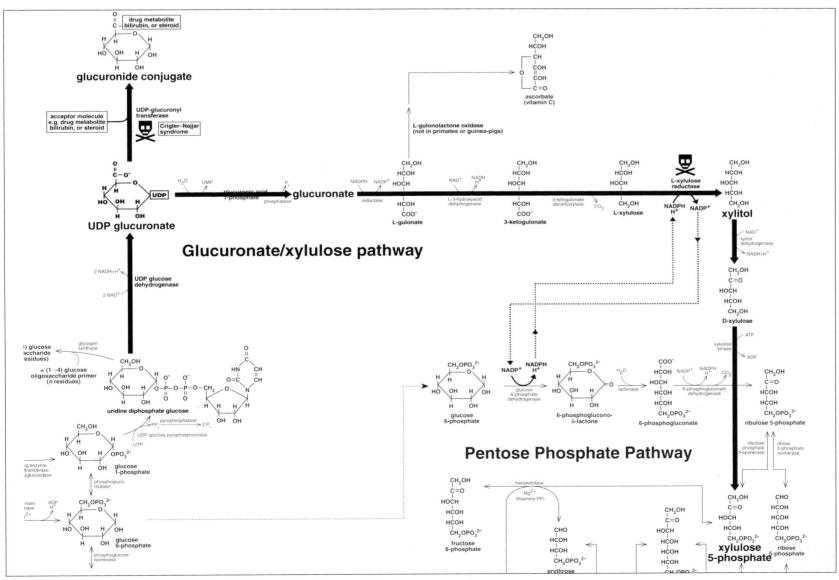

Glucuronate/xylulose pathway

Pentose Phosphate Pathway

Fructose metabolism

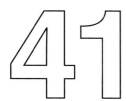

Fructose does not need insulin to enter muscle cells

The average daily intake of fructose in the United Kingdom is around 35–50 g, mainly as the disaccharide sucrose. This is hydrolysed by sucrase in the intestinal cells, forming glucose and fructose. Unlike glucose, however, fructose is able to enter muscle cells and adipocytes in the absence of insulin. Consequently, it has been suggested that intravenous fructose should be given as an energy source in patients suffering major trauma. However, this practice is not favoured currently because of the risk of lactic acidosis, as described below.

Metabolism of fructose by the liver

The liver enzyme **fructokinase** phosphorylates fructose to **fructose 1-phosphate** (Chart 41.1). This is then cleaved by **fructose 1-phosphate aldolase (aldolase B)** to form **dihydroxyacetone phosphate** and **glyceraldehyde**. Glyceraldehyde is then phosphorylated by **triose kinase** to **glyceraldehyde 3-phosphate**. Thus the intermediary metabolites of fructose enter glycolysis as triose phosphates. Their fate now depends on the prevailing metabolic status. However, in the typical circumstances of refeeding after a period of fasting, it is most likely that gluconeogenesis will dominate in the early well-fed state, so that glycogen or glucose will be formed. Alternatively, the substrates could be converted to acetyl CoA and used for fatty acid synthesis.

Metabolism of fructose by muscle

It is likely that the normal dietary quantities of fructose which are presented to the liver in the portal blood will be largely converted to glucose or hepatic glycogen, as described above. Consequently, relatively little fructose will remain for metabolism by muscle. However, if fructose is administered intravenously under experimental conditions, it is metabolized to fructose 6-phosphate by **hexokinase**, since fructokinase is absent from muscle (Chart 41.2). The subsequent fate of this fructose 6-phosphate will depend on the prevailing nutritional status, which will determine whether it is converted to glycogen or used as a respiratory fuel.

Dangers of intravenous fructose

Fructose is metabolized rapidly in humans, having a half-life of 18 minutes. In fact, it disappears from the circulation twice as rapidly as glucose. Although intravenous fructose was once recommended for use in parenteral nutrition, it was not without risk. These dangers accrue because fructose bypasses the regulatory steps which so effectively control glucose catabolism:
1 The entry of fructose into muscle is independent of insulin.
2 Intravenous feeding with large quantities of fructose depletes cellular P_i and lowers the concentration of ATP. Thus phosphofructokinase is deinhibited in muscle and uncontrolled glycolysis from fructose 6-phosphate proceeds.
3 In liver, fructose evades the rate-limiting control mechanism by entering glycolysis as dihydroxyacetone phosphate or glyceraldehyde 3-phosphate, i.e. beyond the regulatory enzyme, phosphofructokinase. The consequence of these effects could be that, in anoxic states, such as result from the shock of severe trauma, rapid intravenous infusion of fructose may cause a massive unregulated flux of metabolites through glycolysis. In extreme circumstances this has led to the production of excessive quantities of lactic acid and precipitated fatal lactic acidosis.

Inborn errors of metabolism
Fructokinase deficiency (essential fructosuria)

This benign condition is due to a congenital absence of fructokinase and is most commonly found in Jewish families. The deficiency means that ingested fructose is limited to metabolism by the hexokinase route only. Consequently, fructose is metabolized much more slowly than usual, so that the blood concentration rises and fructose appears in the urine. Subjects with essential fructosuria have an entirely normal life expectancy.

Fructose 1-phosphate aldolase deficiency (hereditary fructose intolerance)

This serious condition usually presents when an infant is weaned from breast milk on to fructose-containing food. The response to fructose ingestion is a dramatic onset of vomiting and hypoglycaemia within 15–30 minutes. The disorder is due to a deficiency of **fructose 1-phosphate aldolase (aldolase B)**, which results in a massive accumulation of fructose 1-phosphate in the tissues. This process sequesters intracellular inorganic phosphate, and moreover inhibits both glycogen phosphorylase and fructose 1,6-bisphosphate aldolase (aldolase A). The resulting inhibition of glucose production by both glycogenolysis and gluconeogenesis causes the severe hypoglycaemia which is such a serious feature of this condition.

Treatment involves simply avoiding dietary fructose. Patients tend to develop a natural aversion to sweet foods and this usually leads to a complete absence of dental caries. If the condition is not diagnosed and treated, the disease is fatal.

Fructose 1,6-bisphosphatase deficiency

This is a disease caused by impaired gluconeogenesis due to deficiency of this enzyme. It is surprising that, given the strategic importance of fructose 1,6-bisphosphatase in maintaining gluconeogenesis, some patients are relatively unaffected by this disorder. However, in other cases, infants may be hospitalized during the first 6 months of life when the metabolic stress of an infection or fever precipitates hypoglycaemia and lactic acidosis. Although some children with this condition have hepatomegaly and are extremely ill, curiously in other cases this disorder may not be manifested until adult life.

The biochemical pathology results from the stress of trauma or infection provoking a catabolic state in which lipolysis and muscle breakdown combine to produce gluconeogenic amino acids and glycerol. Because gluconeogenesis is inhibited at the fructose 1,6-bisphosphatase reaction, the gluconeogenic metabolites accumulate and form large quantities of lactate. Similarly, ingestion of fructose leads to the formation of lactic acid, precipitating lactic acidosis.

In this condition, glycogenolysis by the liver to release glucose is normal. However, once glycogen is depleted, hypoglycaemia follows due to the failure of gluconeogenesis to maintain glucose homoeostasis. These patients must therefore eat frequent meals to maintain normoglycaemia.

References

Henry R. H. and Crapo P. A., Current issues in fructose metabolism. *Annu Rev Nutr*, **11**, 21–39, 1991.

Prince R. C., Gunson D. E., Leigh J. S. and McDonald G. G., Textbook errors: the predominant form of fructose is a pyranose, not a furanose ring. *TIBS*, 239–40, 1982.

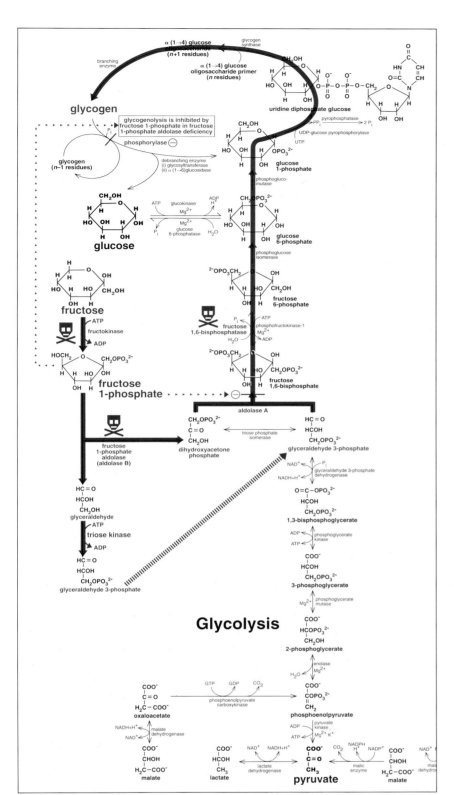

Chart 41.1. Metabolism of fructose to glycogen in liver

Glycolysis

Chart 41.2. Metabolism of fructose in muscle.

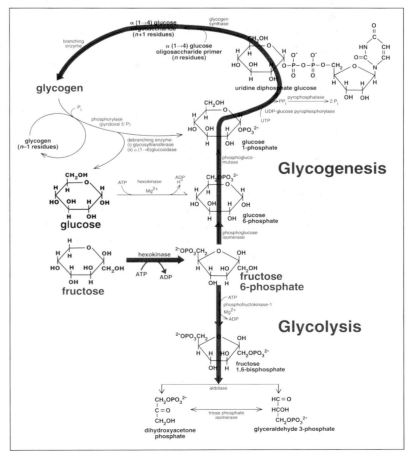

Glycogenesis

Glycolysis

Biochemistry of diabetes

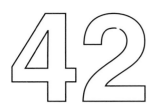

Chart 42 opposite. An overview of intermediary metabolism in diabetes mellitus.

Diagram 42.1. Metabolic relationship of adipose tissue, muscle and liver in diabetes mellitus. (NB: In liver, the bile ducts and canaliculi have been omitted for simplification.)

Hyperglycaemia and ketoacidosis in diabetes

In uncontrolled insulin-dependent diabetes mellitus (IDDM), many metabolic pathways are directed towards the synthesis of glucose and the ketone bodies. This stems from failure of the delicate balance between anabolism and catabolism which is the basis of metabolic homoeostasis in healthy adults.

In diabetes, the anabolic state is impaired because there is insufficient functioning insulin to maintain this balance. Consequently, homoeostasis is redirected towards the catabolic state, and the metabolism of lipids, proteins and carbohydrates is altered as follows.

Metabolism of triacylglycerol in diabetes

In adipose tissue, insulin prevents lipolysis by inhibiting hormone-sensitive lipase (see Chapter 32). In uncontrolled diabetes, therefore, increased lipolysis caused by ACTH and glucagon occurs, so that production of fatty acids and glycerol is increased by up to 300%.

Fatty acid metabolism in diabetes

In the healthy fed state, any fatty acids produced in adipose tissue by lipolysis undergo a cyclic process in which they are re-esterified with glycerol 3-phosphate to reform triacylglycerol (see Chapter 32). In diabetes, this cycle is interrupted due to lack of glycerol 3-phosphate, which is unavailable because it is formed from glucose, which in turn needs insulin to enter the fat cell. Consequently, since re-esterification of the fatty acids is decreased, they are instead released into the blood. Normally, fatty acids would be almost entirely oxidized as a respiratory fuel, especially by the muscles. In diabetes, however, surplus fatty acids are transported to the liver, where they enter the β-oxidation spiral to form acetyl CoA. In the healthy state, this can condense with oxaloacetate for oxidation in Krebs cycle. However, in diabetes oxaloacetate is removed from the mitochondrion for gluconeogenesis, and is in short supply. Consequently, acetyl CoA molecules combine with each other to form 'the ketone bodies', acetoacetate and D-3-hydroxybutyrate (see Chapter 34). Moreover, in the cytosol, acetyl CoA may be diverted in the direction of cholesterol synthesis, which is often increased in diabetes. In severely uncontrolled IDDM, metabolic regulation is deranged and may be associated with a massive production of acetoacetic acid and D-3-hydroxybutyric acid. In serious cases this overwhelms the pH buffering capacity of the blood, causing ketoacidosis.

Glycerol metabolism

The glycerol released from adipose tissue is phosphorylated in the liver by **glycerol kinase** to glycerol 3-phosphate. This is metabolized to glucose, which is released into the blood, contributing to the hyperglycaemia.

Metabolism of protein and amino acids in diabetes

Insulin enhances the uptake of amino acids into muscle from the blood, thus favouring protein synthesis. In diabetes the process is reversed, and muscle protein breaks down to form amino acids. Some of these, particularly alanine, may be released from muscle and used by the liver for gluconeogenesis (see Chapter 18).

Metabolism of glucose and glycogen in diabetes

Insulin is essential to activate the Glu T4 glucose transporters needed for glucose to enter muscle cells and adipocytes. Consequently, in diabetes glucose accumulates in the blood causing hyperglycaemia, while the muscle and fat cells are starved of glucose: a situation described as 'starvation in the midst of plenty'.

Insulin stimulates glycogen synthesis and increases glucokinase activity. In the absence of insulin, glycogen synthesis ceases and glycogenolysis occurs, with glucose being exported from the liver into the blood, once again compounding the hyperglycaemic state.

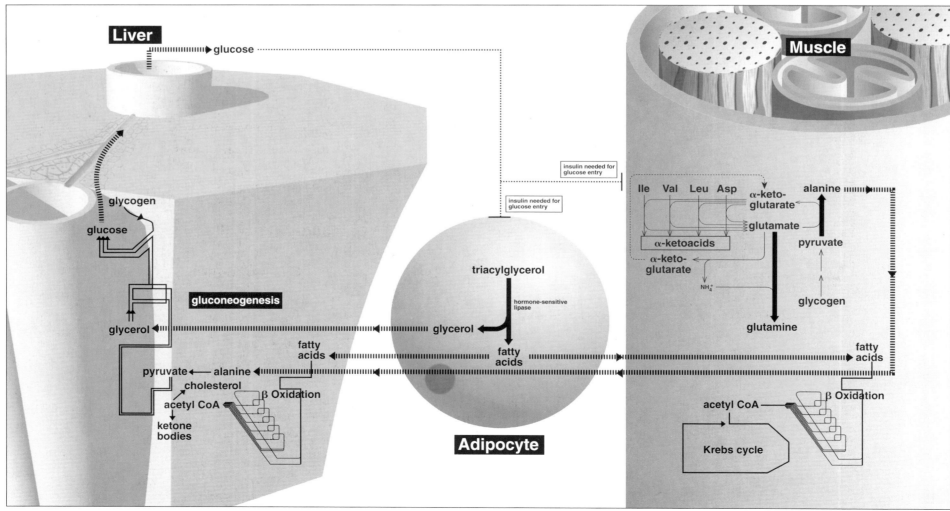

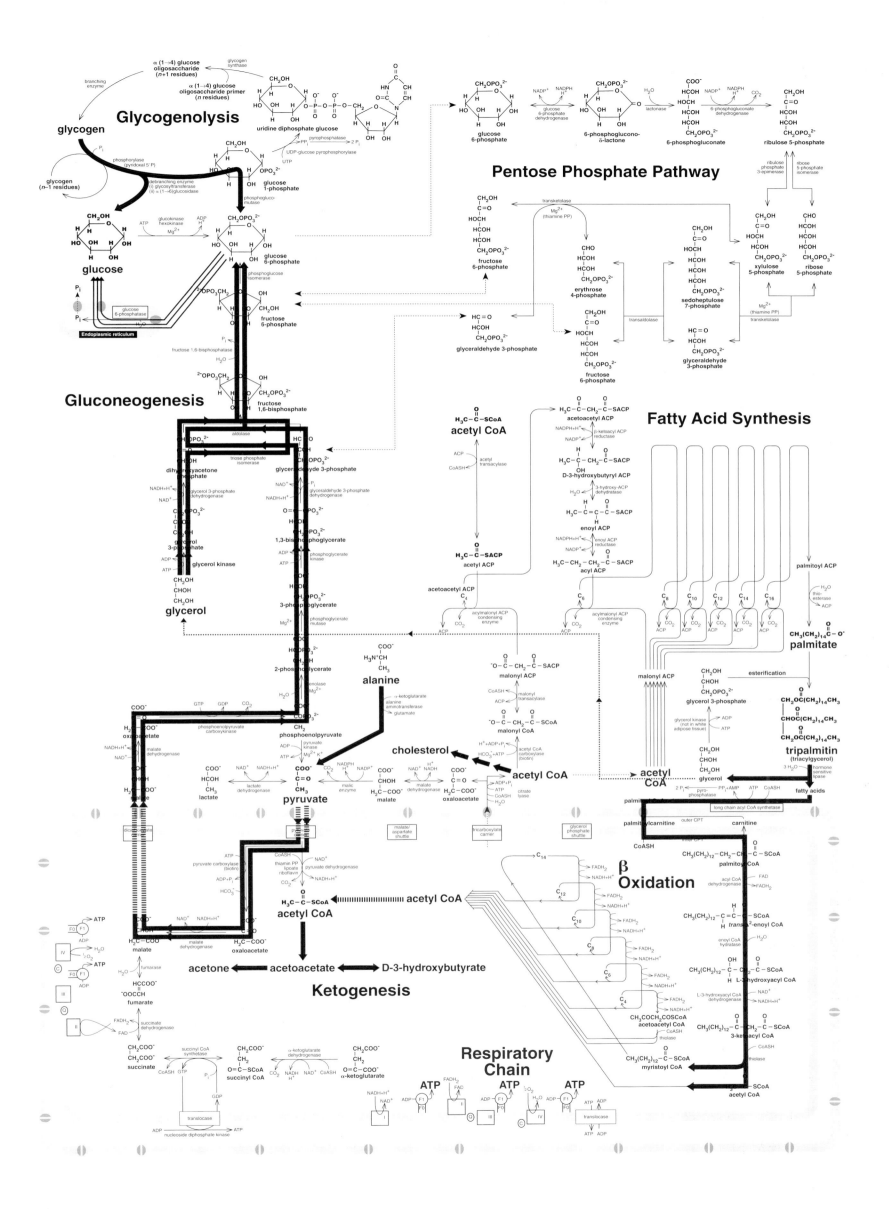

Index

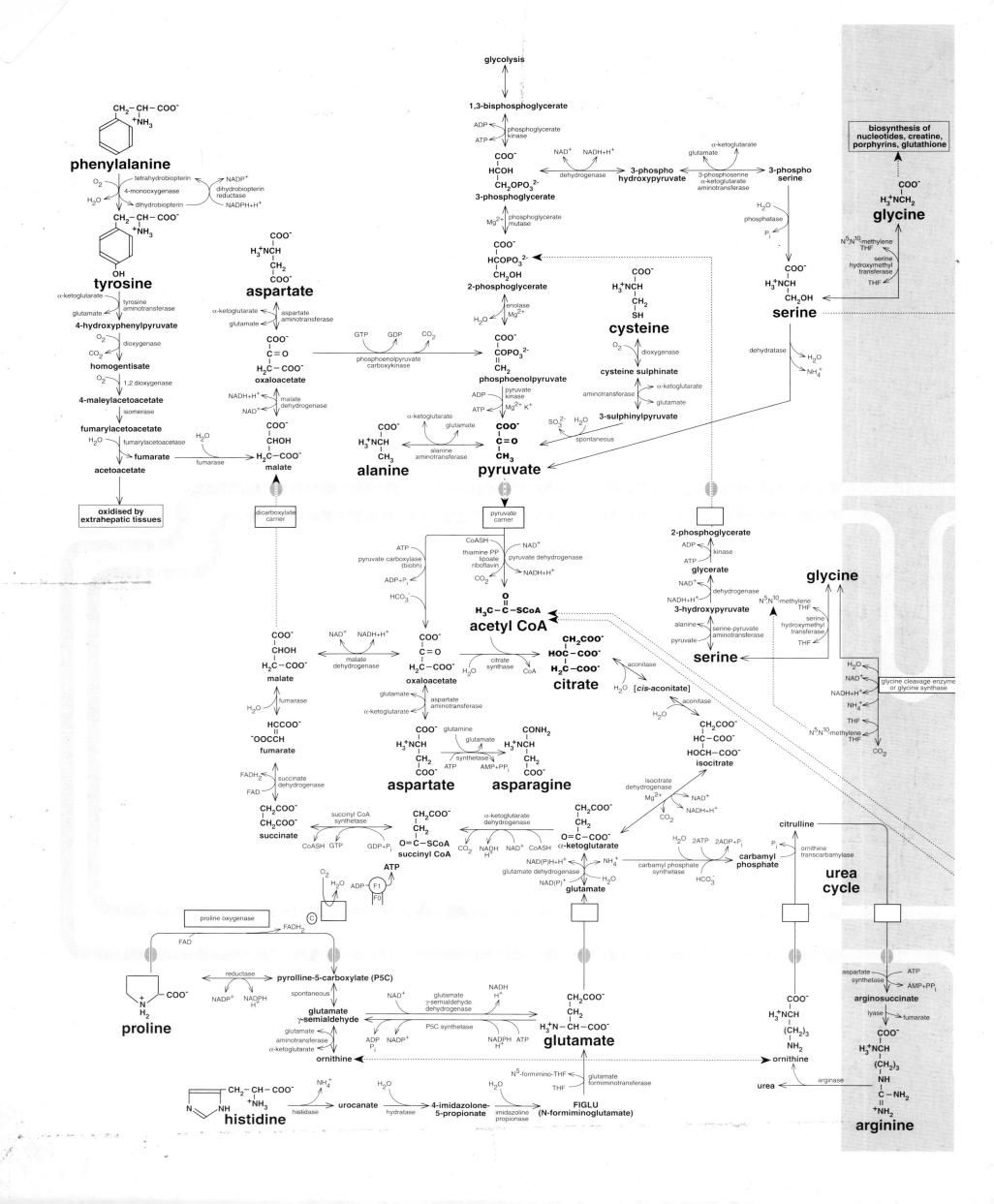